Classical Sanskrit for Everyone

A Guide for Absolute Beginners

Classical Sanskrit for Everyone

A Guide for Absolute Beginners

Malcolm Keating

Hackett Publishing Company, Inc.
Indianapolis/Cambridge

Printed in the United States of America

27 26 25 1 2 3 4 5 6 7

For further information, please address
Hackett Publishing Company, Inc.
P.O. Box 44937
Indianapolis, Indiana 46244-0937

www.hackettpublishing.com

Cover design by Rick Todhunter
Interior design by E. L. Wilson
Composition by Aptara, Inc.

Library of Congress Control Number: 2023952728

ISBN-13: 978-1-64792-190-3 (pbk.)
ISBN-13: 978-1-64792-191-0 (PDF ebook)
ISBN-13: 978-1-64792-195-8 (epub)

The paper used in this publication meets the minimum requirements of American National Standard for Information Sciences—Permanence of Paper for Printed Library Materials, ANSI Z39.48–1984.

∞

Contents

Acknowledgments xi

Grammatical Abbreviations xii

List of Tables xiii

List of Figures xv

How to Use This Book xvi

Introduction xix

1. Writing System and Sounds xx
2. Words xxi
3. Sentences xxii
4. The Lessons xxiii
5. Dictionaries, Grammars, and Other Helpful Tools xxiv

Lesson 1 **1**

1.0 Reading 1

1.1 Vocabulary 3

1.2 Grammar Notes 3

1.2.1 Sanskrit Sound System 3

1.2.2 Sanskrit Writing System 10

1.2.3 Sanskrit Morphology 16

1.3 Putting Everything Together 18

1.4 Further Resources 19

Lesson 2 **21**

2.0 Reading: *Yogasūtra* 1.2 21

2.1 Vocabulary 23

2.2 Grammar Notes 24

2.2.1 *Visarga* Sandhi: Sibilants before Consonants 25

2.2.2 Nominal Sentences 28

2.2.3 Compounds 28

2.2.4 Determinative Compounds 29

2.2.5 Dependent Determinative Compounds 30
2.2.6 Descriptive Compounds 31
2.2.7 Complex Determinative Compounds 31
2.3 Putting Everything Together 34
2.4 About the Reading: Defining Yoga 35

Lesson 3 37
3.0 Reading: *Nyāyabhāṣya* on *Nyāyasūtra* 2.1.32 37
3.1 Vocabulary 39
3.2 Grammar Notes 40
3.2.1 Introduction to Cases: *a*-stem 40
3.2.2 Introduction to Cases: What They Do 43
3.2.3 Verbs: Introduction to 1P and Thematic Verbs 51
3.2.4 The *Repha* 55
3.3 Putting Everything Together 57
3.4 About the Reading: Where There's Smoke, There's Fire 59

Lesson 4 61
4.0 Reading: *Bṛhadāraṇyaka Upaniṣad* 1.4.10 61
4.1 Vocabulary 63
4.2 Grammar Notes 64
4.2.1 Vowel Sandhi: Similar Vowel Combinations 65
4.2.2 Nasal Sandhi: *Anusvāra* 66
4.2.3 Verbs: Introduction to 2P and Athematic Verbs 68
4.2.4 Personal Pronouns: First Person 69
4.3 Putting Everything Together 71
4.4 About the Reading: Ways of Being Brahman 72

Lesson 5 75
5.0 Reading: *Kāmasūtra* 1.2.30 75
5.1 Vocabulary 77
5.2 Grammar Notes 77
5.2.1 *Visarga* Sandhi: Changes before Vowels, Semi-Vowels, and Voiced Consonants 78
5.2.2 The Genitive Case 80

5.2.3 Nasal Sandhi: न् (*n*) to ण् (*ṇ*) 83
5.2.4 Intransitive Verbs: Reminder 84
5.2.5 Adjective Compounds 85
5.2.6 Indeclinables: Negation 87
5.2.7 Prefixes 89
5.3 Putting Everything Together 90
5.4 About the Reading: Romance Is Hard Work 91

Lesson 6 **93**
6.0 Reading: *Chāndogya Upaniṣad* 6.8.7 93
6.1 Vocabulary 95
6.2 Grammar Notes 95
6.2.1 Personal Pronouns: Second Person 96
6.2.2 Demonstrative Pronouns 97
6.2.3 Vowel Sandhi: Dissimilar Vowels 101
6.2.4 Vocative Case 105
6.3 Putting Everything Together 106
6.4 About the Reading: Who Are You? 107

Lesson 7 **111**
7.0 Reading: *Arthaśāstra* 7.9.12 111
7.1 Vocabulary 113
7.2 Grammar Notes 113
7.2.1 Introduction to Relative-Correlative Pairs 114
7.2.2 Verbs in 8P 116
7.2.3 Sandhi: Word-Final Consonants 117
7.3 Putting Everything Together 119
7.4 About the Reading: Friends and Allies 120

Lesson 8 **123**
8.0 Reading: *Hitopadeśa* 1.39 123
8.1 Vocabulary 125
8.2 Grammar Notes 126
8.2.1 Relative-Correlative Pairings: Pronouns 126
8.2.2 Conjunctions, च (*ca*) and वा (*vā*) 130

8.2.3 More about the Instrumental Case 131
8.2.4 Feminine Nouns: *i*-stem 134
8.2.5 Introduction to Sanskrit Verse 135
8.3 Putting Everything Together 136
8.4 About the Reading: Friends, Allies, and Governance 137

Lesson 9 **139**
9.0 Reading: *Mahābhārata* 5.34.10 139
9.1 Vocabulary 141
9.2 Grammar Notes 142
9.2.1 Adjectives 142
9.2.2 Past Passive Participles 146
9.2.3 Future Passive Participles (Gerundives) 149
9.2.4 Comparisons 150
9.2.5 Indeclinables: एव (*eva*), हि (*hi*) 151
9.2.6 Adverbs 153
9.3 Putting Everything Together 154
9.4 About the Reading: Good Advice 156

Lesson 10 **157**
10.0 Reading: *Abhidharmakośabhāṣya* 9 157
10.1 Vocabulary 159
10.2 Grammar Notes 160
10.2.1 Interrogatives 160
10.2.2 Vowel Sandhi: Final ए (*e*), ओ (*o*) 162
10.2.3 Consonant Sandhi: Word-Final Doubling न् (*n*) 164
10.2.4 Verbs: *Ātmanepada* 165
10.2.5 Verbs: Passive Construction 166
10.2.6 Verbs: Optative Mood 168
10.2.7 *an*-Stem Declension: आत्मन् (*ātman*), कर्मन् (*karman*) 169
10.2.8 Syntax: "Carrying Over" Verbs 170
10.3 Putting Everything Together 171
10.4 About the Reading: No Selves, Just *Skandhas* 172

Lesson 11 175

11.0 Reading: *Rājamartaṇḍa* 1.2 175

11.1 Vocabulary 177

11.2 What Commentaries Do 179

11.2.1 Word Division 180

11.2.2 Word Meaning 181

11.2.3 Compound Analysis 185

11.2.4 Sentence Meaning 189

11.2.5 Objections and Replies 191

11.3 Putting Everything Together 193

11.4 About the Reading: Deactivating Mental Activities 195

11.5 Further Resources 196

Lesson 12 197

12.0 Reading: *Raghuvaṃśa* 1.1 197

12.1 Vocabulary 199

12.2 What is Sanskrit Poetry? 200

12.2.1 Kinds of Meter 201

12.2.2 Figures of Speech 208

12.3 Putting Everything Together 213

12.4 About the Reading: Sound and Meaning, Pārvatī and Śiva 216

12.5 Further Resources 217

Lesson 13 219

13.0 Reading: *Bhagavadgītā* 3.14–15 219

13.1 Vocabulary 221

13.2 Lesson Overview 221

13.2.1 Kinds of Translations 222

13.2.2 Translation Conventions 225

13.2.3 Reading Critical Editions 227

13.2.4 Comparing Translations 229

13.3 About the Reading 232

13.4 Further Resources 233

Afterword: Google Translate for Sanskrit 235

Appendix 1: Tables 241

- Sanskrit Writing and Sound System 241
- Vowels 241
- Consonants 242
- Sanskrit "Alphabet" Order for Dictionaries 242
- Numerals 243
- Declensions 244
- Verb Conjugations 250

Appendix 2: Sanskrit Glossary 253

Bibliography 265

Acknowledgments

I will be indebted forever to the scholars and philosophers who introduced me to Sanskrit and honed my skills in reading and translation, whether as formal instructors or reading partners. I have space to mention only a few here from my time at the University of Texas at Austin: Matthew Dasti, Donald Davis, Edeltraud Harzer, Matthew Milligan, Patrick Olivelle, and Stephen Phillips. (None of them, or anyone I thank, are responsible for errors in this book.) I'm also indebted to my students over the last decade or so, whether Sanskrit students or Indian philosophy students, as they have challenged me to improve both my understanding and communication. Bryan W. Van Norden was a source of encouragement throughout this book's writing and even before, in conversations about whether something like his book, *Classical Chinese for Everyone*, was possible for a language like Sanskrit or if a philosopher like me—someone who is not an Indologist or philologist—was the right person to write it. David Buchta kindly reviewed the full draft, patiently discussing important the finer points of Sanskrit grammar with me. He is not culpable for दोष-s but is responsible for many गुण-s. This book would not have come about without Rick Todhunter's skills of persuasion, and I'm grateful that he convinced me in the first place and has been supportive throughout the process. My sister-in-law, Regina Guerrero, read some early drafts of this book from the perspective of a yoga student, keeping me honest about the "for everyone" goal. I'd also like to thank Hackett's production team, especially Elana Rosenthal and Liz Wilson, for their care in bringing this book to fruition—they were attentive to details, from ligature colors to fonts, and patient with my many queries. I'm also grateful to copyeditors Jennifer McBride and Catherine Nelli, whose keen eyes caught errors and inconsistencies that might confuse readers. Nelli's work on the Sanskrit content was invaluable. Finally, my wife, Laura Guerrero, has been immeasurably important for this book's writing.

Grammatical Abbreviations

Grammatical Term	Abbreviation
adjective	adj.
adverb	adv.
ātmanepada	A
compound	cpd.
dative	d.
dual	du.
feminine	fem.
first person	1
genitive	gen.
gerund	gd.
gerundive	gdv.
imperative mood	impv.
indeclinable	indc.
indicative mood	ind.
infinitive	inf.
interrogative	intr.
is equivalent to	=
locative	loc.
masculine	masc.
neuter	neut.
nominative	nom.
noun	n.
numeral	num.
parasmaipada	P
participle	ptp.
particle	ptc.
passive	ps.
past passive particle	ppp.
plural	pl.
prefix	pfx.
preposition	prep.
present tense	pres.
pronoun	pn.
relative	rel.
second person	2
singular	sg.
third person	3
verb	v.
verb root	√

List of Tables

Table 1. Vowels in transliteration 5

Table 2. Guttural consonants in transliteration 6

Table 3. Palatal consonants in transliteration 6

Table 4. Retroflex consonants in transliteration 7

Table 5. Dental consonants in transliteration 7

Table 6. Labial consonants in transliteration 8

Table 7. All sounds in transliteration 8

Table 8. Vowels in Devanāgarī script 12

Table 9. All consonants with Devanāgarī and transliteration 13

Table 10. योग / yoga (*a*-stem noun, masculine gender, nominative case) 17

Table 11. *Visarga* sandhi, sibilants before consonants 27

Table 12. *a*-stem masculine noun (*yoga*), transliteration only 41

Table 13. *a*-stem masculine noun (योग/*yoga*), Devanāgarī only 42

Table 14. *a*-stem neuter (*vana*), transliteration only 43

Table 15. a *a*-stem neuter (वन/*vana*), Devanāgarī only 43

Table 16. Present indicative verb endings, 1P 54

Table 17. Present indicative √भू (*bhū*) (1P) - to be, to exist 55

Table 18. Vowel sandhi, similar vowel combinations 66

Table 19. Nasal sandhi, *anusvāra* 67

Table 20. Present indicative √अस् (*as*) (2P) - to be, to exist 69

Table 21. First-personal pronoun, अस्मद् (*asmad*) 70

Table 22. Consonants in transliteration, with voicing and aspiration 79

Table 23. *Visarga* sandhi before vowels, semi-vowels, and voiced consonants 80

Table 24. *a*-stem neuter, genitive (भद्र/*bhadra*) 82

Table 25. *a*-stem masculine, genitive (योग/*yoga*) 82

Table 26. *an*-stem neuter, genitive (कर्मन्/*karman*) 82
Table 27. Dental and retroflex nasal sandhi 84
Table 28. Second-person pronoun, nominative (युष्मद्/*yuṣmad*) 97
Table 29. First-person pronoun, nominative (अस्मद्/*asmad*) 97
Table 30. Demonstrative pronoun, neuter, nominative/accusative (तद्/*tad*) 100
Table 31. Demonstrative pronoun, neuter, nominative/accusative, (इदम्/*idam*) 100
Table 32. Demonstrative pronoun, neuter, nominative/accusative (एतद्/*etad*) 100
Table 33. Demonstrative pronoun, masculine, nominative/accusative (तद्/*tad*) 100
Table 34. Simple vowels 101
Table 35. Vowel grades according to strength 102
Table 36. Vowel sandhi to corresponding semi-vowel 104
Table 37. Present indicative √कृ (*kṛ*) (8P) - to make, to do, to cause 117
Table 38. Examples of final consonant sandhi, unvoiced and unaspirated 119
Table 39. Relative pronoun, masculine, nominative (यद्/*yad*) 128
Table 40. *a*-stem masculine, instrumental (योग/*yoga*) 132
Table 41. *i*-stem feminine, nominative (प्रकृति/*prakṛti*) 134
Table 42. *ā*-stem feminine, nominative/accusative (कन्या/*kanyā*) 145
Table 43. Final vowel sandhi: ए (*e*), ओ (*o*) 163
Table 44. Consonant sandhi, double final nasal 164
Table 45. Present indicative verb endings, 1A 165
Table 46. Present indicative √भू (*bhū*) (1A) - to be, to exist 166
Table 47. Present optative √भू (*bhū*) (1P) - to be, to exist 169
Table 48. *an*-stem masculine, all forms (आत्मन्/*ātman*) 169
Table 49. *an*-stem neuter, all forms (कर्मन्/*karman*) 170
Table 50. Analysis of *Rājamartaṇḍa* 195

List of Figures

Figure 1. Vocal tract and places of articulation 9

Figure 2. Still from *The Internship* (2013) 10

Figure 3. एतद् (*etad*), इदम् (*idam*), तद् (*tad*) 99

Figure 4. Image of a Jain manuscript, the *Kalpasūtra*, from the Cleveland Museum of Art 223

Figure 5. Sample critical edition, *Bhagavadgītā* 3.14 228

Figure 6. Sample critical edition with annotations, *Bhagavadgītā* 3.14 229

How to Use This Book

Classical Sanskrit for Everyone is designed to give you an orientation to Sanskrit. It isn't a Sanskrit textbook or grammar. It's more like a guided tour of a foreign country. As your tour guide, this book stops to point out and explain important sights along the way, keeping in mind what different audiences might want to see. After all, if you're planning to move to a new country, you might participate in a tour differently than someone on a whirlwind vacation. Below are some general suggestions for getting the most out of the book, depending on your goals. I've identified three general audiences: the Curious (but maybe intimidated), the Yoga Aficionado (or someone similar who knows some Sanskrit), and the Scholar (who has existing language skills). At the beginning of each chapter, I'll identify when sections are especially relevant for these audiences or when you can skip sections to avoid being overwhelmed.

For the Curious

Just focus on reading the lessons and understanding the main ideas.

Don't worry if the sample readings are challenging; keep reading for the big picture.

After reading the lessons, go back and try to work through them more carefully.

For the Yoga Aficionado

Take your time with the pronunciation and script in Lesson 1 to correct any misconceptions.

Write down a list of Sanskrit words you already know and take notes on how the lessons help you understand their meanings and origins.

Make flash cards with the book's vocabulary.

For the Scholar

Use the table of contents to identify lessons on grammatical concepts you're interested in.

For each lesson, after reading, use a grammar listed in the introduction to supplement the book's material.

For Everyone

Look at the afterword on Google Translate to appreciate why learning Sanskrit is still important in the age of artificial intelligence and machine translation.

Skip ahead to Lessons 11, 12, and 13 for general advice on reading commentaries, works in verse, critical editions, and translations.

Bookmark the appendices to refer to as you read.

Look at the website, https://hackettpublishing.com/sanskrit-for-everyone-support, for translations of each lesson's readings—but try to work them out yourself first.

Introduction

Sanskrit is one of the world's oldest languages. It is the language of the *Yogasūtra*, the *Mahābhārata*, the *Rāmāyaṇa*, and the *Bhagavadgītā*. (We'll talk about the marks in those words soon.) These texts are well-known as part of what we now call "Hinduism," but Sanskrit was not only a language for Hindu texts. Buddhists and Jains wrote in Sanskrit, too. As an ancient language, Sanskrit is connected to many other languages in a family known as "Indo-European." English, as part of this Indo-European family, has words that bear striking similarities to Sanskrit words, given the languages' shared linguistic origins—take, for instance, "father" and *pitṛ*, "mother" and *mātṛ*. Modern English has borrowed some words without any change. Today, people talk about karma and dharma, nirvana and yoga, without batting an eye. But although Sanskrit happily loans modern English speakers a smattering of vocabulary, it parts with expertise less easily. It is grammatically complex and challenging for novices to learn.

When I was a beginning Sanskrit student, one of my instructors told the class about a king who tried to learn Sanskrit. The king's wife had spoken to him in the language, and when he couldn't understand her, he felt humiliated. This king asked one potential instructor, a court minister, how quickly he could learn Sanskrit. (Kings are busy, after all.) The answer was that it usually took twelve years of dedicated focus, but this minister could help the king do it in just six years! Eventually, the king gets the help of the goddess Sarasvatī, along with a different instructor, and he learns Sanskrit in a mere six months.[1] My teacher's moral? Without divine intervention, six years is an impressively fast time to learn, so we burgeoning Sanskritists shouldn't give up after just two or three!

1. This story is told in Somadeva's *Kathāsaritsāgara*. In it, the court minister who teaches the king also vows to give up all spoken language if he succeeds in his task. He does, but as a result of his vow and some other adventures, he writes a brilliant book of stories, so all eventually ends well.

This book introduces absolute beginners to the main contours of Classical Sanskrit, but unlike the king's ministers, it doesn't aim to make you fluent enough to have conversations. (In fact, it doesn't teach you to speak Sanskrit at all.) And, unlike my university instructor, it doesn't presume you want to be a Sanskritist in six years or twelve. *Its goal is to explain and illustrate some of the main features of the language*, along with one of the most common scripts in which it's written. It does not pretend to be a Sanskrit textbook—other excellent ones already exist, referenced throughout. Instead, this is a readable *orientation* to the language. You'll learn to read the script, understand the way sentences are put together, and be able to look up words in a dictionary. Then, if you want to learn more, you'll know where to start.

So, let's begin by introducing you to the main skills you need to read Sanskrit: the ability to interpret the writing system and sounds, the ability to identify words and their meanings, and the ability to understand sentences. (Scholars familiar with these concepts may wish to skip to section 5 below.)

1. Writing System and Sounds

First, you need to recognize the letters on the page. This is a matter of learning a *script*, which is a writing system. For instance, you're reading English, which is written in Roman script and is basically the same script as French and Spanish. In contrast, the Russian and Ukrainian languages use the Cyrillic script. Instead of writing "A, B, C, D . . . ," someone speaking these languages would learn to write "А, Б, В, Г . . ." Here's a Russian word printed in Cyrillic: язык. (It's a word that means "language.") Each symbol stands for a particular letter. If you wanted to learn Russian or Ukrainian, you'd need to learn this script. Sanskrit has been written in a range of scripts, but in this book, we'll learn Devanāgarī, which starts in a sequence we'll discuss later: "अ आ इ ई . . ." (It's the same script used for modern Hindi.)

You'll also want to learn Roman *transliteration*. Transliteration lets us represent the words in one script using another script. The Russian word язык is transliterated into the Roman script as *yazyk*. A Roman equivalent represents each Cyrillic letter: *y* represents я, *a* represents з, etc. Similarly, the Sanskrit word शब्द ("language") is transliterated as śabda. Symbols like श् correspond to Roman letters like ś. The ´ mark over the "s" and the little bars across the vowels in *Devanāgarī* are essential for reading Sanskrit because they tell us how to pronounce the words (which we'll turn to soon). You need to learn to pair these written symbols with the sounds that they make because this is how languages communicate meaning. I belly up to a bar and order a beer—I don't belly up to a beer and order a bar. The system of sounds that makes up a language is called its *phonology*.

2. Words

When we read a language, we aren't just reading groups of letters representing sounds. We're reading sentences, which are made up of words. So, you'll need to learn how words change in context, or *morphology*. The "morph" in "morphology" means change. Like Morpheus in *The Matrix* or the heroes of the *Mighty Morphin Power Rangers*, words can change their forms depending on what they're doing. In English, for instance, we often make a word plural by adding "-s" at the end: "She reads a book" becomes "She reads books." English students must learn which words take "-s" at the end, which take "-es," and which don't change when plural, like "deer."

Sanskrit, too, has a system of morphology to learn. But Sanskrit morphology goes beyond just communicating number. From a word's form, we can learn a lot more information than whether there is one rabbit or two. And morphology doesn't just apply to nouns, like "book" and "deer," but also to verbs, like "read" and "leap."

Running through all of the above is vocabulary! This is often what people think of when they think of learning a language: adding a stock of new words to their memory. Learning vocabulary will help you read new sentences, of course, as well as have concrete examples of how words change in context.

3. Sentences

Beyond morphology is *syntax*, how we put words together to form sentences. In English, syntax is dependent on word order. That means whether Buttercup likes Roberta or Roberta likes Buttercup depends on what order the words appear in the sentences. Sanskrit, in contrast, is much less concerned with the order of words. This means that the morphology of words—how they are formed—can tell us who is the *subject* and who is the *object* of an action, in other words, *who* likes *whom*.

But there is one place where word order is important. This is a communicatively powerful aspect of Sanskrit: *compounds*. Again, using English as a comparison, most of us are familiar with some compounds, like "blackbird" and "cupcake." To see why word order is important here, in English as in Sanskrit, try flipping the words within the compound: "birdblack" and "cakecup." These are very different! Probably you'd put a cupcake *in* a cakecup, and "birdblack" sounds like the name of a paint color. Sanskrit uses compounds, too, but these compounds can become very lengthy, to the point where they are essentially complete sentences.

For all of the categories above—writing system, phonology, morphology, and syntax—there are lots of potential rules and exceptions we could cover. However, in this book, I'll introduce you to some important general principles, give you a few key examples, and illustrate them with some actual Sanskrit texts. This means you'll be reading Sanskrit by the end of the book. It doesn't mean you will be able to pick up just any Sanskrit text and read it—but you'll have the tools to start filling gaps in your knowledge.

4. The Lessons

In the following pages, I introduce you to major principles in Sanskrit by giving examples from actual Sanskrit texts. Each lesson starts with an overview of what you'll learn and includes (1) an example reading, (2) a vocabulary list, (3) grammar notes, and (4) supplemental discussions.

Example readings. The readings are written in both Devanāgarī and Roman transliteration. Try reading the Devanāgarī script first before the Roman transliteration. Make sure you understand what parts of the script the transliteration represents as you go. It's a good idea to practice writing out the reading as well. You might even try memorizing some readings—many are famous and quite short.

Vocabulary lists. The book presents the words as you'd find them in a dictionary—their stem or root form. Because of the importance of morphology in Sanskrit, as we saw above, it's important to learn the fundamental form of a word before it acquires new endings or changes in other ways. As with the readings, the vocabulary is presented in Devanāgarī and Roman. Each vocabulary term has grammatical information in abbreviation. You can find a list of these abbreviations at the beginning of the book. Each new term is followed by a succinct definition, focusing on its meaning as used in the reading.

Grammar notes. Sections on grammar explain key principles of Sanskrit grammar to help you with the reading. These notes are highly generalized and do not attempt to be comprehensive. For readers interested in a deeper dive—and there are much deeper waters to explore!—you can check out the footnotes, where I make some qualifications and cite further resources. (I've called them "pandit points," a tip of the hat to Bryan W. Van Norden's "nerd notes" in his book *Classical Chinese for Everyone.*) Along the way I include sample sentences that illustrate the key concepts in the lessons. They are easier than the main readings, which are taken from actual Classical Sanskrit texts.

Supplemental discussions. The end of each lesson contains more information about the content of the reading, interesting linguistic facts about Sanskrit, and references for further reading.

5. Dictionaries, Grammars, and Other Helpful Tools

The resources below will be helpful if you decide to go further in learning Sanskrit or wish to look up more details about grammar or word meanings. Looking words up in a Sanskrit dictionary requires knowing the order of the Sanskrit "alphabet," which most dictionaries have in their introductory pages. It also requires recognizing what the fundamental form of a word is since, as we've seen, Sanskrit words change their form quite a lot. This book will help you understand the basic principles of using dictionaries well.

Textbooks

Deshpande, Madhav. M. *Saṃskṛta-Subodinī: A Sanskrit Primer*. Ann Arbor: University of Michigan Press, 1999. Along with the Goldmans' textbook (below), this is one of the most commonly used introductory Sanskrit textbooks. Desphande proceeds more slowly than the Goldmans do.

Egenes, Thomas. *Introduction to Sanskrit*. Part 1, 3rd rev. ed. Delhi: Motilal Banarsidass, 2003. Given the difficulty of Sanskrit, this is probably the best guide for students wanting to learn on their own. It takes students even more piecemeal and stepwise than Deshpande.

Goldman, Robert P. and Sally J. Sutherland Goldman. *Devavāṇīpraveśikā: An Introduction to the Sanskrit Language*. Delhi: Motilal Banarasidas, 2011. While a difficult book to learn from independently, it can be a useful reference guide along with the other grammars below. It includes adapted passages from the *Rāmāyaṇa* for practice.

Ruppel, A. M. *The Cambridge Introduction to Sanskrit*. Cambridge: Cambridge University Press, 2017. This textbook is paired with an online support page, and plenty of videos to help you learn how to write Devanāgarī and pronounce Sanskrit sounds (https://www.cambridge-sanskrit.org).

Dictionaries

All three of the below dictionaries are commonly used for Sanskrit:

Apte, Vaman Shivaram. *Revised and Enlarged Edition of Prin. V. S. Apte's The Practical Sanskrit-English Dictionary*. Poona: Prasad Prakashan, 1957–1959.

MacDonell, Arthur Anthony. *A Practical Sanskrit Dictionary with Transliteration, Accentuation, and Etymological Analysis Throughout*. London: Oxford University Press, 1929.

Monier-Williams, Monier. *A Sanskrit-English Dictionary*. Delhi: Motilal Banarsidass, 1963. First published 1899.

Grammars

MacDonell, Arthur Anthony. *A Sanskrit Grammar for Students*. 3rd ed. Oxford: Oxford University Press, 1927. A concise guide to Sanskrit grammar with helpful charts.

Whitney, William D. *The Roots, Verb-Forms, and Primary Derivatives of the Sanskrit Language*. Delhi: Motilal Banarsidass, 2006. First published 1887. A reference guide to the basic forms of words and their transformational patterns.

Whitney, William D. *Sanskrit Grammar Including Both the Classical Language, and the Older Dialects, of Veda and Brahmana*. Cambridge, MA: Harvard University Press, 1889. This detailed, classic grammar is old enough to be available free on Wikisource, at https://en.wikisource.org/wiki/Sanskrit_Grammar_(Whitney), which makes it an excellent searchable reference.

Online Resources

A number of universities now host online resources. These include:

The Institute of Indology and Tamil Studies. 2023. "Cologne Digital Sanskrit Dictionaries." Cologne University. Last modified December 19, 2023. https://sanskrit-lexicon.uni-koeln.de/. Version 2.7.29 of this site has thirty-eight dictionaries, along with grammatical tools useful for the analysis of noun declensions and verb conjugations.

Sanskrit at the University of Chicago. n.d. University of Chicago (website). Accessed December 26, 2023. http://www.prakrit.info/vrddhi/resources/. Designed and maintained by Andrew Ollett of the University of Chicago, this site is a collection of resources aimed at introductory-level learners. It includes lessons, annotated readings, and links to resources.

University of British Columbia Sanskrit Learning Tools. n.d. University of British Columbia (website). Accessed December 26, 2023. https://ubcsanskrit.ca/. UBC hosts lessons and readings with color-coded charts. (Some require a login.)

South Asia Institute. n.d. Sanskrit at the University of Texas at Austin (website). Accessed January 19, 2024. https://sites.utexas.edu/sanskrit/. The site has student-focused resources as well as lesson plans for instructors, along with transcriptions of texts in polity and law (*dharmaśāstra*).

Beyond university-affiliated websites, there are others:

The Sanskrit Dictionary. n.d. Accessed December 26, 2023. https://sanskritdictionary.com. This site aggregates a number of dictionaries into a single search. It also hosts a searchable version of the grammarian Pāṇini's *Eight Chapters*, a tool for splitting sandhi (which we'll talk about in the second lesson), along with a fun Sandhi Invaders video game.

The Sanskrit Library. 2015. https://sanskritlibrary.org/. The site includes digital texts as well as resources for learning Sanskrit, such as the "Conjunct Explorer," a self-test for learning the more than 1,400 conjuncts that appear in Devanāgarī. The Library also offers courses.

Lesson 1

योगः

yogaḥ

Points of Interest For

The Curious: Use the tables in this lesson as a reference; just skim the details about pronunciation for now.

The Yoga Aficionado: Look at Figure 1 as you read through how to pronounce sounds.

The Scholar: Be sure to try the self-tests in 1.2.1 and 1.2.2.

1.1 Vocabulary

Devanāgarī	Transliteration	Part of Speech	Translation
योग	yoga	masc. n.	discipline, method, practice

Note: The vocabulary lists include abbreviations for important pieces of information. These are listed before the lessons. Here, "masc." means "masculine," and "n." means "noun" (see Grammatical Abbreviations). We'll talk about this below.

1.2 Grammar Notes

KEY POINTS: You'll learn how to read the Devanāgarī script, the basics of how to pronounce Sanskrit, and how to read and write some common Sanskrit words.

1.2.1 Sanskrit Sound System

KEY POINT: The tables in this section include Sanskrit sounds in transliteration, paired with English words to help you learn how to pronounce Sanskrit sounds. Table 6 summarizes the pronunciation and points out transliterations you might misunderstand.

By the end of this lesson, you'll be able to read, write, and pronounce the very common word above, written in Devanāgarī. And in addition, you'll have some more general knowledge about language. That's because a wonderful thing about learning Sanskrit is that you'll start paying attention to the kinds of sounds you make in whatever language you speak. Instead of an alphabet in what seems like a random order (why is A the first letter and B the second, and who put Z all the way at the end?), the

Sanskrit language orders its component sounds—and corresponding written symbols—in terms of where the sounds are made in your mouth and throat.[1] These points of articulation are used to group vowels, consonants, and what are known as *semi-vowels* because they're in between vowels and consonants. There is a lot I could say about these sounds, but instead of giving you all the information in the introduction here, I will share it with you as we go when it helps you with the reading. The consonants can be pronounced roughly like English sounds without too much of a problem, though I'll flag some differences. The vowels are also close to English pronunciations, though some differences between them are crucial, especially the difference between long and short. So, let's start with them.

Vowels

Vowels marked with a *macron* (the ¯ symbol) are long and held a bit longer than their corresponding short vowel. Below I will approximate pronunciation using some example words spoken with a "standard" American accent. The italicized and bolded part of the word is an approximation for pronunciation. For more precise representations, look at the online resources listed at the end of the Introduction.[2]

1. Pandit point: Here's the book's first "Pandit Point"—footnotes that will share more detailed information for readers who want it. A "pandit" (in English, sometimes also "pundit") or a *paṇḍita* (पण्डित) in Sanskrit is a learned person. Written Sanskrit doesn't use an alphabet, strictly speaking, but an "abugida" (also known as an "alphasyllabary"), where characters represent a consonant and a vowel together.

2. If you are already familiar with the International Phonetic Alphabet (IPA), you can look up a table of Sanskrit sounds and their IPA equivalents online for a more precise guide. The Wikipedia entry for Sanskrit currently has such a guide under the section "Pronunciation" (https://en.wikipedia.org/wiki/Sanskrit#Pronunciation). You can also hear the IPA spoken at its official website (https://www.internationalphoneticalphabet.org). However, since most people who aren't linguists don't know the IPA and teaching it in addition to teaching Sanskrit would be too much, this book won't use the system.

Table 1. Vowels in transliteration

Short Vowel	Long Vowel
a - b***u***t	ā - b***aw***dy
i - b***i***t	ī - b***ee***
u - p***u***t	ū - p***oo***l
ṛ - ***r***ig	ṝ - ***r***ig[3]
ḷ - al***lr***ight	ḹ - al***lr***ight
e - b***ai***t	ai - b***i***te
o - r***o***te	au - r***ou***nd

With just this information, you can take a pop quiz about how to pronounce a very common Sanskrit word related to the first word in our lesson: *namaste*.[4] Based on the spelling, what does it most closely rhyme with? (a) "Naw, I'mma stay!" (b) "Bahamas, hey!" (c) "Um, us, yay!" Check the end of the Lesson for the right answer.

Now that you've learned to correctly pronounce one of the most frequently mispronounced Sanskrit words, let's look at consonants and semi-vowels. I will introduce them to you in groups based on where in your mouth and throat you pronounce them. That will be important later on.[5] For now, just focus on the major ideas about pronunciation.

---

3. Pandit point: This is a very uncommon vowel, though it exists. It's a longer version of ऋ (*ṛ*). The vowel ऌ (*ḷ*) is extremely uncommon, and ॡ (*ḹ*) is a hypothetical form that Sanskrit grammars include for symmetry. We won't worry about these three vowels in this book. That's why they're in gray. One other point: you will sometimes see ऋ transliterated as *r̥* and ऌ as *l̥*. That is because other Indic scripts (used to write languages like Bengali, Punjabi, etc.) have different sets of sounds, and *ṛ* and *ḷ* are used for other sounds in those languages (in a transliteration system known as ISO 15919). If the transliteration is of Sanskrit, you don't need to worry about any difference between the dot *ṛ* and the small circle *r̥*—they both represent ऋ.

4. Pandit point: This word means "hello" and is also an ordinary greeting in Hindi.

5. You can look at Appendix 1 for a more detailed table of the sounds and their symbols. It includes a concept we'll talk about later, voicing. (See Lesson 5.)

Look at Figure 1 to help you understand where your tongue will be placed when you make the sounds.

Guttural

The *guttural* sounds are formed in the back of your throat, at the velum. Consonants with an "h" after them are pronounced with a little puff of air, known as *aspiration*. (Say "skunk" and then "kite" and listen for the difference in the sound after the "k." The second has aspiration, which I've represented with the symbol +A.)

Table 2. Guttural consonants in transliteration

-A	+A	-A	+A	-A	+A
k - s**k**unk	kh - **k**ite	g - **g**ate	gh - lo**gh**ouse	ṅ - si**ng**	h - **h**ay

Palatal

These sounds are *palatal*, formed with your tongue against the roof of your mouth. Notice that the transliteration c is pronounced "ch" as in "chew," not a soft "c" as in "nice" or a hard "c" as in "consider."

Table 3. Palatal consonants in transliteration

-A	+A	-A	+A	-A	-A	+A
c - **ch**ew	ch - **ch**alk	j - **j**eep	jh - he**dge**hog	ñ - i**n**ch	y - **y**ellow	ś - **sh**irt

Retroflex

These sounds are *retroflex*, formed with your tongue curled back near the front of your mouth. English speakers often struggle with these because we tend to put our tongue at the alveolar ridge (see Figure 1). But no Sanskrit sounds do this! Avoid this part of your mouth. The tongue should be curled just behind it when pronouncing these sounds. (Because English lacks some of these sounds, the examples are the same as the dentals below.)

Table 4. Retroflex consonants in transliteration

-A	+A	-A	+A	-A	-A	+A
ṭ - s**t**eer	ṭh - **t**ear	ḍ - **d**eer	ḍh - re**dh**ead	ṇ - de**n**t	r - d**r**ama	ṣ - ru**sh**

Dental

Take the word *dental* seriously for these sounds. They're formed with your tongue touching your teeth. Again, avoid the alveolar ridge. The best way to learn these sounds is by listening to audio: you can find links in the Online Resources at the end of the Introduction.

Table 5. Dental consonants in transliteration

-A	+A	-A	+A	-A	-A	+A
t - s**t**eer	th - **t**ear	d - **d**eer	dh - re**dh**ead	n - de**n**t	l - **l**ook	s - **s**traw

Labial

These sounds are *labial*, formed with your lips pressed slightly together. Note that the "v" sound is somewhere in between a "w" and a "v"—if you find your top teeth touching your bottom lip, you're not quite there. Try again, with just air through your lips.

Table 6. Labial consonants in transliteration

-A	+A	-A	+A	-A	-A
p - s**p**in	ph - **p**in	b - **b**in	bh - a**bh**or	m - **m**um	v - **w**ay

We'll talk more about pronunciation as we go, so don't worry too much about these details just yet. (Think of this lesson as a helpful reference.)

Table 7 shows all the consonants in the order we saw above. Notice that I have divided the rows up to distinguish what are called *semi-vowels* from the consonants. A semi-vowel's sound is between a consonant and a vowel. Each row but the first has *sibilants*, or "s" sounds. The sound *ha* gets its own column. The entries with an asterisk * are ones English speakers commonly mispronounce, so this is a good point to check your understanding by going back to the earlier tables if you're uncertain.

Table 7. All sounds in transliteration

Point of Articulation	**Consonants**					**Semi-Vowels**	**Sibilants**	***ha***
Aspiration	- A	+ A	- A	+ A	- A	- A	+ A	+ A
Guttural	ka	kha	ga	gha	ṅa*			ha
Palatal	ca*	cha	ja	jha	ña*	ya	śa*	
Retroflex	ṭa	ṭha*	ḍa	ḍha	ṇa*	ra	ṣa*	
Dental	ta	tha*	da	dha	na	la	sa	
Labial	pa	pha*	ba	bha	ma	va		

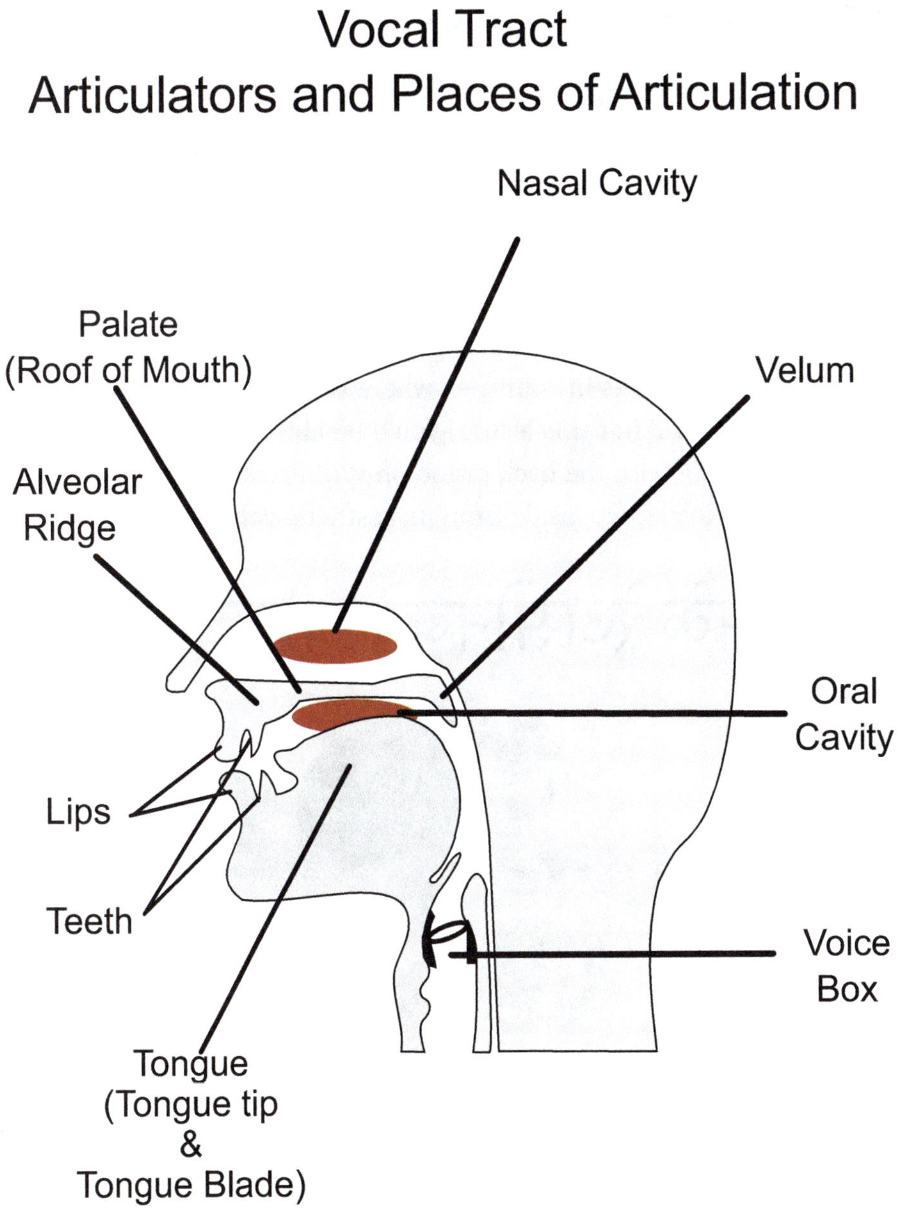

Figure 1. Vocal tract and places of articulation. Source: Tavin, Wikimedia.org, https://commons.wikimedia.org/wiki/File:Tract.svg

1.2.2 Sanskrit Writing System

> **KEY POINT:** The Devanāgarī writing system represents a single sound with multiple forms, depending on its relationship with surrounding sounds.

Another reason that this book is an orientation to Sanskrit and not a complete introduction is because the writing system is complex. This is not only a challenge for learning the language but also for tattoo artists and their clients in countries where the script isn't familiar, like the United States. After this lesson, you'll be able to understand what's so terribly wrong with the neck tattoo on Will Ferrell's character in the 2013 film *The Internship*, aside from its aesthetic value:

मके रेअसोनब्ले चोइचेस

Figure 2. Still from *The Internship* (2013)

Take a close look at it and come back after you've read the rest of the lesson! See if you can (1) sound it out using the charts above, and (2) identify any mistakes. Answers at the end.

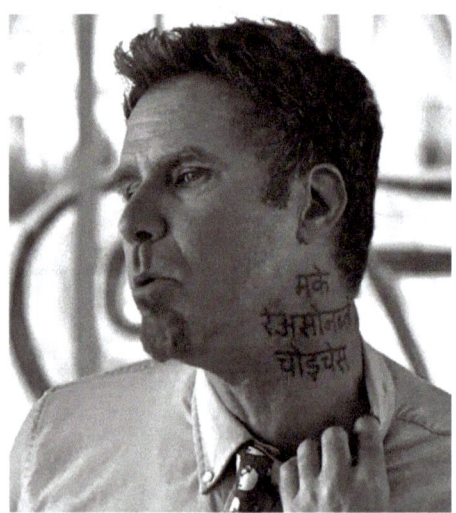

Below is an introduction to the main written symbols, but it isn't comprehensive. Here's our first vowel, which we learned above, "a," written in Devanāgarī:

अ

Sanskrit symbols are written left to right, top to bottom.[6] (See the list of resources at the end of the Introduction for help on how to write them.) You'll notice what looks like the numeral "3" is attached to a long vertical bar with a horizontal line, and the vertical bar has its own short horizontal bar at the top. All of the symbols have this horizontal line, which it looks like they hang from.[7] And most have the long vertical bar, though some of them have a shorter version, which looks like a little peg, or they just hang down. So in writing these, you're learning different marks in relationship to these two bars. Table 8 shows the vowels we learned earlier:

---

6. Pandit point: I will assiduously avoid using the word "letter" in this book because it can confuse people into thinking that क in Devanāgarī is the same thing as "k." It's not, as we'll see. But note that other books may use the word "letter." And you might be wondering what the names of the Sanskrit sounds are since English speakers learn how to say the alphabet: "A," "B," "C," etc. For most of them, in Sanskrit, you would simply pronounce the sound and add the word कार (*kāra*) afterward. So अ (*a*) is *a-kāra*. There are only a few exceptions, which we'll learn.

7. Pandit point: Typographers call the location of the horizontal line the *headline*, and a whole vocabulary has developed to describe the parts of these symbols. For those interested in appreciating the graphic components of Devanāgarī, Saxena (n.d.) is a helpful online article. For those more interested in the details, see Naik's (1971) massive three-volume work on the Devanāgarī script cited in Saxena.

Table 8. Vowels in Devanāgarī script

Short Vowel	Long Vowel
अ a - b**u**t	आ ā - b***aw***dy
इ i - b**i**t	ई ī - *bee*
उ u - p**u**t	ऊ ū - p**oo**l
ऋ ṛ - **r**ig	ॠ ṝ - **r**ig
ऌ ḷ - al**lr**ight	ॡ ḹ - al**lr**ight
ए e - b***ai***t	ऐ ai - b**i**te
ओ o - r**o**te	औ au - r**ou**nd

You may notice a pattern—the long vowels add one extra component, like another vertical bar in the case of अ and आ or a small mark at the top in the other cases, like इ and ई. The order of entries in a Sanskrit dictionary moves horizontally across Table 8—first comes अ (*a*), then आ (*ā*), after these इ (*i*) and ई (*ī*), and so on.

Now, let's look at consonants and semi-vowels. One important point: the written symbol in the script doesn't just represent the consonant, like "k" in the Roman script. Rather, it includes the vowel sound "a" directly after it. For instance, this symbol

क

is pronounced "ka" as in "***ca***thedral." All of the consonant symbols below are like this, which is why I include the vowel in the transliteration next to them. If we want to just represent "k" without the vowel, we'd stop the vowel sound from occurring with a little stop mark under the consonant:[8]

---

8. Pandit point: This is one difference with Hindi. If you hear people talking about "dharm" and not "dharma" or "yog" instead of "yoga," it's because, in Hindi, there is no assumption of that vowel sound afterward. Neither pronunciation is right or wrong—they're just different languages! The little mark is called a *virāma*, by the way.

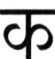

क्

Table 9 shows the consonants written with their dependent vowel in the order we saw above.

Table 9. All consonants with Devanāgarī and transliteration

Point of Articulation	Consonants					Semi-Vowels	Sibilants	ह
Aspiration	- A	+ A	- A	+ A	- A	- A	+ A	+ A
Guttural	क ka	ख kha	ग ga	घ gha	ङ ṅa			ह ha
Palatal	च ca	छ cha	ज ja	झ jha	ञ ña	य ya	श śa	
Retroflex	ट ṭa	ठ ṭha	ड ḍa	ढ ḍha	ण ṇa	र ra	ष ṣa	
Dental	त ta	थ tha	द da	ध dha	न na	ल la	स sa	
Labial	प pa	फ pha	ब ba	भ bha	म ma	व va		

Phew! Now you have a guide to the main sounds and their representations in Sanskrit. We'll talk about others along the way, and in Appendix 2, you have an entire list, along with a guide to their order in a dictionary, but you're now almost ready to get started. There are just two more things to know about the writing system: dependent/independent vowels and consonant conjunctions.

Dependent and independent vowels

> **KEY POINT:** You will never see अ (*a*) or the other vowels appear in their independent form in the middle of a word.

Above, we learned what vowels look like when they're *independent*, that is, when they're hanging out by themselves. So, at the start of a word, you'll see them appear like अ or इ. But we also learned that vowels can be *dependent*, like the "a" after "k" as in क (*ka*). The vowel अ (*a*) is so dependent that it disappears when it is next to another symbol! In fact, all of our vowels change in their dependent form, and these changes are essential to learn so you can recognize them when they show up in the middle or at the end of words.

Here are a few that will be important for our first reading. You can look at the full chart in Appendix 1, and I'll introduce others along the way:

कि ki, को ko,
के ke, कू kū, कृ kṛ

Notice that the vowels appear in a few different places. The short "i" appears in front of the "k" in कि (*ki*), while the "o" appears after in को (*ko*). The "e" is a small mark on top in के (*ke*), and the "ū" and "ṛ" both typically appear underneath: कू (*kū*), कृ (*kṛ*).[9] These are the four main places that you'll see a consonant modified with vowels. While at first, seeing the "i" in front of क may feel strange and look like it should read "ik," over time, you'll naturally think of कि as *ki*, I promise!

Consonant conjunctions

The last important transformation that happens in the writing system is a *consonant conjunct*, and that's, as you probably have guessed, what happens when two consonants run into each other. In this book, we will not learn them all. There are a lot! As you get more comfortable with the script, you will probably be able to figure out new conjuncts, but I will always help you with them, at a minimum, by providing a transliteration. Here's one:

9. Pandit point: Sometimes you'll see "ū" and "u" pop up in other places, like रू (*rū*) and रु (*ru*). You will have transliterations throughout the book to help you learn these combinations.

श्च

If you look back at the consonants in Table 9, you might guess the bottom symbol. It's च (*ca*). And, if you remember that Sanskrit is written from top to bottom, left to right, you might also guess that the squiggle at the top comes before च (*ca*), and you'd be right! This is our friend, श् (*ś*), which you can find at the end of the palatal row above. Notice that in the last sentence, I made sure to put the stop mark underneath श् (*ś*) since the symbol is directly in contact with च (*ca*)—there's no vowel in between them. Conjuncts are common, and they signal that there is no intervening vowel. So, we'd read श्च as "śca." (In the next lesson we'll see why this strange-sounding combination is important.) You've also just learned another Sanskrit word: च (*ca*). This is the word for "and," which we'll encounter again in our readings. Another common conjunct is when त् (*t*) comes into contact with त (*ta*).

त्त

You might be getting the sense of a pattern now! Conjuncts often squish the first symbol into space above the second symbol. Here, the doubled "t" is like what we'd find in the word चित्त (*citta*), meaning "thought."[10] This word combines what you learned about dependent vowels, चि (*ci*), and conjuncts, त्त (*tta*). Can you guess what the conjunct below is? It's *tr*icky, but give it a *try*!

त्र

10. You may wonder what the rule is for italicizing Sanskrit words in this book. Sanskrit words that have been adopted in other languages, like "sandhi" and "yoga" aren't italicized. Words in parentheses that gloss the Devanāgarī are, like योग (*yoga*). For ease of reading, examples and readings with long sentences in Sanskrit do not use italics.

1.2.3 Sanskrit Morphology

KEY POINT: Sanskrit words change form to communicate information about their precise meaning in a sentence.

After spending so much time on individual symbols and their sounds, you might wonder if we'll ever get around to words. That's the focus of *morphology*, how words change form to convey different information. I'll explain the basic ideas throughout the book, so here, let me just introduce one main idea we'll work with: cases.

Sanskrit is a case-declined language, which means that its nouns change their form, or *decline*, to communicate the role they play in a sentence, understood by a grammatical category known as a *case*. In English, we understand these roles by a combination of word order and prepositions:

1. He gives the sword *to* the queen.
2. The queen slays the lion *with* a sword.

In the first sentence, the fact that "the queen" comes after "to" tells us she is the one who receives the sword. In the second, the fact that "the sword" comes after "with" tells us it is the instrument of her slaying. But in Sanskrit, the basic form of the words "queen" and "sword" would change in sentences (1) and (2). The words could appear just about anywhere in the sentence, and we'd know how they're being used because changes in form tell us what case a word is in—we wouldn't need any prepositions either.

There are eight cases in Sanskrit, which are associated with different roles a noun can play, like *subject*, *object*, or *instrument*.[11] This idea will become clearer as you read, but compare the cases to roles an actor plays. The same actor in multiple films might change their role by

11. Pandit point: Some books will say there are *seven* cases because the vocative doesn't count as its own case. We'll talk about the vocative in Lesson 6, and I discuss the number of cases in note 10 in Lesson 3.

changing hair color, using different facial expressions, or wearing different costumes. Like an actor, a Sanskrit word takes on different forms for its different roles. As I'm sure you've had your fill of charts, I won't introduce you to these roles—and cases—here. These will appear in Lesson 3. Instead, I'll give you an example of what one noun looks like in one case. Take the word we're looking at in this lesson, which refers to a kind of mental discipline:

योगः

In the vocabulary list, I've introduced this word to you in its *stem* form. That is the form you'd look up in a dictionary. Notice what's different:

योग

In the stem form, योग (*yoga*), the word doesn't have an ending. If I want to use योग (*yoga*) as the subject of a sentence, I add an ending that communicates its case and its number. For instance, the form you see above is the *nominative*. That form communicates how many yogas there are. In English, we use singular and plural: there is a yoga or many yogas. But in Sanskrit, we can identify words as dual and say there are two yogas. So, we can decline योग (*yoga*) as follows:

Table 10. योग / yoga (*a*-stem noun, masculine gender, nominative case)

Singular	Dual	Plural
योगः yogaḥ (a yoga)	योगौ yogau (two yogas)	योगाः yogāḥ (many yogas)

Notice that the singular and plural have what looks like a colon after them—this is a symbol for a little puff of air that lightly echoes the vowel before, like *yoga-*^{hah}, and you'll see it a lot. In the following lessons, you'll learn about the other cases and the different patterns (or declensions) that words can have, and why. The pattern for योग (*yoga*) is for a *masculine* noun ending in अ (*a*). In a grammatical context, this doesn't mean that yoga is particularly macho or related to masculine people. Grammatical *gender* is just a way of distinguishing between the morphological patterns we discussed earlier.

1.3 Putting Everything Together

Now, we can go back to the word at the beginning of the lesson and say it out loud. It's pronounced *yoga*-^{hah}, with that little puff of breath at the end.[12] That means it is declined and means (one single) "yoga." You now know that in Devanāgarī, "yoga" is spelled योग, and this is its stem form, which you'd look up in a dictionary. You also understand that ो (*o*) is the dependent form of ओ (*o*), and that ग (*ga*) is pronounced like "g**u**t" and not "g**a**ther." Finally, in Sanskrit, a single word can be a complete sentence! In many contexts, when a word is declined in the nominative, meaning it is the subject, we can mentally insert the verb "to be." From the single word योगः (*yogaḥ*), we can understand the full sentence, "There is yoga."[13] But what is योग (*yoga*)? That will be the topic of our next lesson, in which we'll read a definition of yoga by the philosopher Patañjali (पतञ्जलि).

12. Pandit point: To refine your pronunciation, try to avoid making the *visarga* a full syllable, like "yoga-hah." In Lesson 12 on meter, we'll see why that's important. The *visarga* is really just a little breath of air.

13. Pandit point: This is why you'll often see translators use square brackets—they want to be sure you know that the words "There is" aren't being translated from equivalent Sanskrit words. So someone might write, "[There is] yoga." But that doesn't mean that the translator is just guessing or adding meanings willy-nilly. See Lesson 13 for more about translations.

1.4 Further Resources

For learning Devanāgarī:

Ashtanga Yoga. 2023. “The Devangari Game—Learn How to Read Sanskrit Texts in the Original Version.” https://www.ashtangayoga.info/philosophy/sanskrit-and-devanagari/devanagari-learning-game/.

Sanskrit Library. 2015. “Conjuct Explorer.” https://sanskritlibrary.org/conjunctExplorer.html.

Self-Quiz Answers

namaste (नमस्ते) The answer to the pop quiz is (c). Most English-speakers badly mispronounce this word, at least as it should be pronounced in Sanskrit. Both “a” sounds are short, not long.

मके रेअसोनब्ले चोइचेस is an attempted transliteration of “make reasonable choices.” Someone has tried to replace each Roman letter with its Devanāgarī equivalent. But if we read this as we would Sanskrit, there are problems: (1) notice the independent forms of dependent vowels in two places (अ, इ) makes it spelled incorrectly, and (2) the sounds don’t work—for instance, the “a” in “make” is not the same as मके, which would be pronounced more like “muh-kay.” Sounding this out, we would have “muh-kay ray-uh-so-nuh-blay cho-ee-chay-sa.” Certainly not a reasonable choice.

Lesson 2

Reading: Yogasūtra 1.2

योगश् चित्तवृत्तिनिरोधः ॥

yogaś cittavṛttinirodhaḥ.

Points of Interest For

The Curious: Pay attention to the English examples of sandhi in 2.2.1 and compounds in 2.2.3–7.

The Yoga Aficionado: Look for Pandit Points about yoga and the discussion of *namaste* in 2.2.1.

The Scholar: Look for Pandit Points about Sanskrit grammatical theory.

2.1 Vocabulary

Note that vocabulary lists will include not only vocabulary from the main reading but also from examples throughout the lesson. The grammatical details for many of these forms will wait until later lessons, but they're included so you can begin to recognize them (and commit them to memory if you'd like). Pay attention to whether the word is given to you in its basic stem form or in a declined form. If it's declined, it will include abbreviations for the case, like "nom." for nominative.

Devanāgarī	Transliteration	Part of Speech	Translation
।, ॥	.	punctuation mark known as a *daṇḍa*: singly, acts as a period; doubly, it acts as a full stop at the end of a verse or section	
१	1	num.	one (other numerals are in Appendix 1)
आसन	āsana	neut. n.	posture, pose
च	ca	indc.	and
चित्त	citta	neut. n.	thought, awareness
टीका	ṭīkā	fem. nom. sg. n.	gloss, notes (a kind of commentary)
तत्	tat	neut. nom. sg. pn.	it, that
ते	te	2 pn. d.	for you, to you
देव	deva	masc. n.	god, deity
नमः	namaḥ	neut. nom. sg. n.	honor

निरोध	nirodha	masc. n.	stopping, cessation, restraint
नील	nīla	adj.	dark color, dark blue
पङ्क	paṅka	neut. n.	mud, dirt
पुरुष	puruṣa	masc. n.	person, man
पुस्तक	pustaka	neut. n.	book
महा-	mahā-	adj., cpd. form of महत् (mahat)	great, noble
योग	yoga	masc. n.	discipline, method, practice
राजा	rājā	masc. nom. sg. n.	king, leader
वृत्ति	vṛtti	fem. n.	movement, activity
शिष्य	śiṣya	masc. n.	student
सारथि	sārathi	masc. n.	charioteer
सूत्र	sūtra	neut. n.	short saying, aphorism; thread

2.2 Grammar Notes

KEY POINTS: You'll learn about sandhi, how to read nominal sentences, how to read compounds (the determinative), and the definition of yoga according to Patañjali.

For our first reading, we are looking at a *sūtra* text. The word *sūtra* literally means "thread," and a *sūtra* text is a strand of thoughts connected together. These kinds of texts were meant to be memorized in their entirety—and still are today. In this lesson, we're looking at the *Yogasūtra*, which could be translated as the *Aphorisms on Discipline* and is written by the philosopher Patañjali.[1] It's probably from the first-century Common Era (CE), though, like many early Sanskrit works, scholars disagree about the date. If you go online looking for a translation of this text (and I suggest you don't, not yet!) you will find many. That divergence is because of a few things we'll learn about in this lesson.

First, words in Sanskrit can have a wide range of meanings. Sometimes, a word can even mean both one thing and its opposite. Second, compound words can be understood legitimately in a few different ways. Often, context will clarify what the author means, but sometimes authors intentionally use these ambiguities, especially in poetry (see Lesson 12). The *Yogasūtra* is well-known and influential and provides a chance to see three crucial features of Sanskrit in action: sound combination, nominal sentences, and compounds.

2.2.1 *Visarga* Sandhi: Sibilants before Consonants

> **KEY POINT:** Systematic changes in sound, known as sandhi (or *saṃdhi*), are incorporated into a word's spelling in Sanskrit.

The first word in our reading looks different than the forms of योग (*yoga*) we learned in Lesson 1. However, योगश् (*yogaś*) is, in fact, the nominative singular form of the masculine noun we learned. When योग is the subject of a sentence, it is in the nominative, which means it ends with a *visarga*, as in योगः (*yogaḥ*). When that breath-like sound[2] comes

1. Pandit point: Traditionally, the author of the *Yogasūtra* is identified as the same person who wrote a famous grammatical work, the *Mahābhāṣya*. Contemporary scholars aren't sure about this identity, as it was not until the eleventh century that this connection was made, and we don't have any independent evidence one way or the other.

2. Pandit point: This sound is called a "post-vocalic aspiration." Early Sanskrit grammarians characterized these and other ideas in a highly sophisticated manner in early works, such as Pāṇini's *Aṣṭādhyāyī* or *Eight Chapters*. It may upset some purists, but in this book, I will not do much with Pāṇini's grammar. However, if you are interested in the topic, check out Staal (2003). The *Eight Chapters* is available digitally online at http://sanskritdictionary.com/panini/.

into contact with the च् (c) at the beginning of the next word, it changes. This change is called *sandhi*. "Sandhi" is a Sanskrit word that means "combination" or "conjunction."[3] This phenomenon happens in many languages, but what is unusual about Sanskrit is that it systematically represents these changes in writing.

Take the phrase "fun and games" as said in American English. Almost no one will pronounce the "d" at the end of "and." Rather, they'll say something closer to "fun anggames" as the "d" assimilates to the "g" and is run together with "games." (Try it yourself!) However, no one spells the phrase this way. In Sanskrit, however, these systematic transformations are put into writing. That means that you would read the equivalent of "fun anggames" in print and need to recognize that "ang" is "and" rather than a strange new word.

Here, we see sandhi, where the *visarga* becomes a श् (ś).[4] The light sound of the *visarga* often transforms when it comes into contact with other sounds. You will see a lot of *visarga* sandhi. How the sound changes depends on what vowel precedes it and what sound comes after. You can find materials online and in textbooks that will help you learn all the permutations. For our example, we see a *visarga* change to an "s" sound, a sibilant. There are three kinds of sibilants the *visarga* changes to when it comes into contact with three kinds of consonants, shown in Table 11.[5]

---

3. Pandit point: Strictly speaking, the word would be spelled संधि (*saṃdhi*) in Sanskrit, but it's become a loanword in English. In this book, I spell it the way you'll often see it.

4. Pandit point: There is a further change in printed Devanāgarī, which we'll talk about in Lesson 7. In conjunction with चि (*ci*), the श् is printed as श्चि (*ści*).

5. Pandit point: Two other initial sounds generate this change, the aspirated versions of the dentals in Table 11. Since words beginning with these sounds are rare, I have omitted them. For fun, go back to Lesson 1 to find the missing initial sounds, then look at a Sanskrit dictionary to see how many words begin with them.

Table 11. *Visarga* sandhi, sibilants before consonants

Final *Visarga*	Initial Sound		Final Sibilant	Initial Sound	Example
गः (-gaḥ)	च (c-)		गश् (-gaś)	च (c-)	yogaḥ ca → yogaś ca[6] योगः च → योगश् च
गः (-gaḥ)	छ (ch-)	→	गश् (-gaś)	छ (ch-)	yogaḥ chedaḥ → yogaś chedaḥ योगः छेदः → योगश् छेदः
गः (-gaḥ)	ट (ṭ-)		गष् (-gaṣ)	ट (ṭ-)	yogaḥ ṭīkā → yogaṣ ṭīkā योगः टीका → योगष् टीका
गः (-gaḥ)	त (t-)		गस् (-gas)	त (t-)	yogaḥ tat → yogas tat योगः तत् → योगस् तत्

Now that you understand this pattern, you also can appreciate another common Sanskrit word: नमस्ते (*namaste*). This word is two words, नमः (*namaḥ*) and ते (*te*), which, after sandhi, combine into नमस् (*namas*) + ते (*te*). They are printed together and have become a single word in modern Hindi. You will notice that the right vertical line in the sibilant symbol स् (*s*) disappears in this consonant conjunct:

स् + त = स्त

The word नमः (*namaḥ*) means "salutation" or "honor," and ते (*te*) is a form of the personal pronoun for "you," which we'll talk about in Lesson 6. Together, the phrase means "honor to you."[7]

---

6. Pandit point: In printed Devanāgarī, there is a further change, which we'll discuss in Lesson 7. In conjunction with चि (*ci*), the श् (*ś*) is printed as श्चि (*ści*). The other sibilants also change form in printed Devanāgarī. See if you can figure out what these conjunctions are: ष्ट, ष्ठ.

7. Pandit point: Although you'll find many explanations of the supposed deeper meanings of this expression, in its most basic, literal meaning, it is a greeting. In modern India, as a loan word in Hindi, it just means "hello." Depending on the context, this can mean anything from "hi" to something more weighty, as when it's used to address gods

2.2.2 Nominal Sentences

> **KEY POINT:** Sanskrit sentences often do not need an explicit verb form of "to be," such as "is" or "are."

In Sanskrit, we can choose to write sentences without verbs. These are called *nominal* sentences because they consist only of nouns that are equated with each other, or are in apposition. For instance, suppose I want to say, "The tree is an oak." I could express it just by saying, "Tree oak." That's the typical word order in Sanskrit.

Pattern

noun1 noun2

noun1 is the noun2

Example

Yoga cessation.

Yoga is the cessation.

Nominal sentences are fairly common in Sanskrit, especially since nouns (and adjectives—see Lesson 9) carry much information just by their form. We'll look at sentences with verbs in future lessons.

2.2.3 Compounds

This lesson introduces you to a concept many textbooks save for much later: compounds. However, because so many Sanskrit words are compounds, we'll talk about this idea early. Understanding compounds lets us use a greater variety of Sanskrit texts in our lessons. English has compounds, too, like "blackbird," "cupcake," and "redcoat" (referring

---

like Agni in the *Ṛgveda*. Unlike many analyses you may find online or hear in a yoga studio, there is no mention of "light" in this word.

to a British soldier).[8] Compounds allow authors to communicate a lot of information in a short space because hearers interpret the relationship between the component parts—it doesn't need to be spelled out. A blackbird is a bird that is black, a cupcake is a cake the size of a cup, and a redcoat is a person who wears a coat that is red. In what follows, don't worry too much about the technical terms for the compounds—focus on understanding the patterns.

2.2.4 Determinative Compounds

KEY POINT: Sanskrit compounds typically involve relationships of equivalence or dependence between the final word and the other words in the compound.

One important kind of compound is a *determinative compound*.[9] These compounds end with a noun, which we call the *head* of the compound. The other words in the compound have a specific relationship to that head noun, which the reader understands through context and typically not through case endings. This relationship can be equivalence or something else, like possession.

8. Pandit point: Compounds in English are often, but not always, joined together as a single word. Sometimes, compound nouns are separated by a space (as in "fire truck"). Determining whether two English words (a noun and its modifier) are in compound is not straightforward and depends on stress patterns and whether the elements can be modified. See Downing (2015, 396–97).

9. Pandit point: All of these kinds of compounds, and indeed, all of the grammatical terms, have Sanskrit names. I will not use them in this book, although many Sanskrit books do. In addition to being an entryway into Sanskrit grammatical theory, they're valuable terms because they are often *autological* (also called *homological*). That means they illustrate the property they refer to. In English: "word" is a word. In Sanskrit, the word for a determinative compound is *tatpuruṣa*. The first word, *tat*, is an undeclined pronoun that we understand in context to mean "of him" or "his." The second word, *puruṣa*, means "servant" or "person." So, the compound means "his servant," which illustrates how these compounds work. The term *tatpuruṣa* is a *tatpuruṣa*.

Another way to put this: we usually cannot identify the case of the words in the compound by their spelling. Remember that the case of योगः (*yogaḥ*) is nominative and we can tell because of the final *visarga* (go back to 2.2.1). In contrast, in compounds, we have to think about the *meaning* of the words. The same goes for number: the ending of a noun in Sanskrit tells us if there is one, two, or many of that thing. But in a compound, that ending is lopped off, so it depends on context whether we should understand the compounded word in the singular, dual, or plural. Below are two kinds of these compounds. Lesson 3 will introduce you to the case relationships in more detail.

2.2.5 Dependent Determinative Compounds

One very common relationship between words is *possession*. Without using a compound, we might communicate that an object belongs to something or someone by putting it in a particular case called the *genitive*. If we wanted to say in Sanskrit, "This book belongs to the student," we'd mark the word "student" (शिष्य, *śiṣya*) so that it means "*of* the student." (You'll see how this works in Lesson 3.) But we can communicate this same idea in a compound by putting the noun "student" directly in front of the noun "book" without changing the spelling from the stem form that we learned about in the introduction to this Lesson.

Pattern

noun2-noun1 = the noun1 of noun2

Example

शिष्यपुस्तकम्

śiṣyapustakam

a book (*pustakam*) of a student (*śiṣya*); a student's book

If I'm talking about a book that a student owns, I might say शिष्यपुस्तकम् (*śiṣyapustakam*) to mean "student-book," or "a book *that belongs to* a student." These kinds of determinative compounds are called *dependent* determinative compounds because the other words depend on the head noun in various ways. Possession is one such dependence relationship, and we'll see there can be other relationships, too. Just about any relationship other than equivalence will work.

2.2.6 Descriptive Compounds

A compound expressing equivalence tells us that something *is* something else. We also call these *descriptive* compounds because the head noun is described by the earlier word.

Pattern
noun2-noun1 = the noun1 that is noun2

Example
महाराज
mahārāja
the king (*rāja*) which is great (*mahā*); the great king

We can't distinguish between the descriptive and dependent determinative compounds just by looking at their form. They won't have special endings or spelling changes. Instead, we need to think about the relationship between the head noun (the final word in the compound, like "king") and the other words (like "great"). Saying that the king *belongs to* great, for instance, doesn't make sense, nor does saying that the book *is* a student.

2.2.7 Complex Determinative Compounds

We can create longer compounds, too. We just add another word before the compounded word. Then that new word has its own relationship to whatever the previous part of the compound refers to. And that relationship doesn't need to be the same as the first, nor does it need to be possession. In future lessons, we'll get more precise about these relationships and how they relate to the cases. At this point, try thinking about the *meaning* of the words and what kinds of relationships they might have. Then, make an educated guess. For example, we might have a combination of descriptive and dependent determinative compounds:

Pattern

noun3-noun2-noun1 = the noun1 of the noun2 which is a noun3

Example

नीलपङ्कज

nīlapaṅkaja

what is born (*ja*) from the mud (*paṅka*), which is blue (*nīla*)

This compound, which means "blue lotus," is made up of a dependent determinative compound, "mud-born" or "born from the mud," a term for a lotus, in combination with an adjective, "blue." The adjective is in the same case as "mud-born," so "blue-(mud-born)" is a descriptive compound. The point here is to see that this compound involves multiple relationships.

Now, let's put everything together with one last example, which is a bit silly but will illustrate the points. Take the compounds "half-shell-hero" and "teenage-mutant-ninja-turtle." What is the relationship between the component parts? Notice that we can start from the head nouns, "turtle" and "hero," and work backward to unpack the relationships pairwise. I'll use brackets around the pairs of words to illustrate:

Example

teenage-mutant-ninja-turtle

[ninja-turtle] = a turtle which is a ninja

mutant-[ninja-turtle] = a ninja-turtle which is a mutant

teenage-[mutant-[ninja-turtle]] = a mutant-ninja-turtle which is teenage

In this first example, the head noun ("turtle") is in apposition with the other members of the compound. (Here, "mutant" could be understood as an adjective or a noun.) Of course, if you aren't familiar with the Saturday morning cartoon of the same name, you'd be forgiven for thinking that maybe this is a turtle that *belongs* to a ninja. This very ambiguity makes attention to context important and is why interpreting older texts can be difficult. To see how a compound should be understood in context, try inserting the phrase "which is" between the two words if you think it might involve equivalence, that is, apposition. If you think it is a dependent determinative compound, try out different prepositions, like "in," "of," "at," "from," "for," "by," and so on, between the words.

Location is another common relationship between component parts. And sometimes you can't just work back to front.

Example

half-shell-hero

[half-shell] = half of a shell

[half-shell]-hero = hero inside of half of a shell

In our second compound, notice that the relationship between "hero" and "half-shell" is not equivalence. The half-shell is not the hero! The turtle *inside* of the half-shell is the hero. Again, the way to know this is to try out different understandings. Inserting "which is" between "shell" and "hero" doesn't make sense: "The hero which is a shell."

Now, we can combine our understanding of compounds and nominal sentences to approximate our first reading's structure:

Example

The teenage-mutant-ninja-turtle half-shell-hero.

This nominal sentence has no verb, but if we were to "translate" it into ordinary English, it would read, "The teenage mutant ninja turtle *is* a hero in a half shell." At this point, go back to the sentence from the *Yogasūtra* and try reading it again before moving on.

2.3 Putting Everything Together

> योगश् चित्तवृत्तिनिरोधः ।
>
> yogaś cittavṛttinirodhaḥ.

To read this sentence, start from the front:

1. Recognize part of the word योग- (*yoga-*) and notice the sibilant श् (*ś*). This suggests that the word योगश् (*yogaś*) may once have ended with a *visarga* -गः (*-gaḥ*) and changed. That means the first word is in the nominative case, making it the subject of our sentence.
2. Notice that the ending to the long string of words is -धः (*-dhaḥ*). We learned above that words in the masculine nominative singular, a-stem form, end this way. So, this expression refers to one thing. It is in the same case as योगश् (*yogaś*). Since Sanskrit sentences can be made of two words in apposition, योगश् (*yogaś*) is in apposition with the rest of the sentence:

   योगश् (is) चित्तवृत्तिनिरोधः ।

   Discipline is *cittavṛttinirodhaḥ*.
3. Now consider what the compound expresses. Recognize that the head noun is निरोधः (*nirodaḥ*), which means "restraining," and start there:

योगश् (is) चित्तवृत्ति**निरोधः** ।

Discipline is *cittavṛtti-***nirodhaḥ**.

Discipline is *cittavṛtti-***restraining.**

The restraining could be in apposition with *cittavṛtti*, or there could be a dependence relation:

Discipline is the restraining that is *cittavṛtti*.

Discipline is the restraining of *cittavṛtti*.

To decide, you must examine the compound more closely.

4. Go back to the vocabulary list to help you see that there are two other members of the compound:

   योगश् (is) **चित्तवृत्ति**निरोधः ।

   Discipline is ***citta-vṛtti****-nirodhaḥ*.

   Discipline is **thought-activity**-restraining.

Now, you can consider the relationships among all three members of the compound. Are they in apposition, like "mutant-turtle," or do they have other relationships, like possession, location, etc.? One way to work this out is to consider each pair in turn and think about potential meanings. Don't forget, too, that the members of the compound can be singular, dual, or plural. The restraining is singular, but how many things are being restrained (activity or activities, a thought or many thoughts)? You can check your work with the translations online and in Lesson 11, where a translation is printed along with Bhoja's commentary.

2.4 About the Reading: Defining Yoga

In our reading, Patañjali defines yoga as a kind of discipline involving cessation or restraint. While today, the word "yoga" is often associated with bodily movement, known in Sanskrit as आसन (*āsana*), this is not the main subject of the *Yogasūtra*. Rather, it focuses on mental and ethical *disciplines*. That's because the word योग (*yoga*) is derived from another Sanskrit word, युज् (*yuj*), which originally referred to yoking or restraining an animal, as when you yoke two oxen together on a farm. It's from this original meaning that the extended meaning of "discipline" as self-restraint emerges.

Unlike most modern people, Patañjali doesn't use "thought" (चित्त, *citta*) for only intellectual actions, like when you do math problems or, more broadly, just think. For him, it refers to a range of psychological features such as our will, perception, and more—but for Patañjali, these features aren't part of our deepest selves. Our self is instead a silent, inactive witness to the hurdy-gurdy cause-and-effect world. The philosophical tradition of Yoga, with a capital "Y," refers to the tradition following Patañjali, using his text as a starting point for understanding the self and universe. For more on this text, see Bryant (2015). But in the little "y" sense of "yoga," many Indian and South Asian philosophers do yoga since they have their own specific disciplines for training the body and mind.[10]

---

10. When talking about topics like "Indian philosophy," it's important to recognize that the modern nation-state of India has political boundaries that only date to the middle of the twentieth century. The geographic range of premodern Sanskrit literature was much broader: depending on the time period, it was found in modern-day Afghanistan, Bangladesh, Bhutan, Nepal, Pakistan, Tibet, Sri Lanka, and beyond, throughout Southeast and East Asia.

Lesson 3

Reading: Nyāyabhāṣya on Nyāyasūtra 2.1.32

धूमप्रत्यक्षदर्शनात्
अग्नौ अनुमानम् भवति ।

dhūmapratyakṣadarśanāt agnau anumānam bhavati.

Points of Interest For

The Curious: If not reading Devanāgarī script yet, skip 3.2.4; focus on understanding the cases (as usual, look at tables and example sentences).

The Yoga Aficionado: Read 3.4 for an introduction to philosophers who pair yoga with reasoning.

The Scholar: Pay attention to the typical Sanskrit word order in 3.2.2.

3.1 Vocabulary

Devanāgarī	Transliteration	Part of Speech	Translation
अग्नौ	agnau	masc. loc. sg. n.	about fire; in fire
अनुमान	anumāna	neut. n.	an inference
अश्व	aśva	masc. n.	horse
गच्छति	gacchati	v. (1P), 3 sg. v. from √gam	he/she/it travels, goes
ग्राम	grāma	masc. n.	village, town
दर्शन	darśana	neut. n.	experience, observation
धर्म	dharma	masc. n.	righteousness, religion, ethical principle, law, rule
धूम	dhūma	masc. n.	smoke
न्याय	nyāya	masc. n.	right reason, rule; name of philosophical tradition
प्रत्यक्ष	pratyakṣa	neut. n.	perception
बुद्ध	buddha	masc. n.	the Buddha (lit., "enlightened one" or "awakened one")
√भू	√bhū	v. (1P)	to be, to exist (see 3.2.2 to understand the √ symbol)
राज्य	rājya	neut. n.	kingdom
राम	rāma	masc. n., proper name	Rāma
वन	vana	neut. n.	forest
सागर	sāgara	masc. n.	ocean

3.2 Grammar Notes

> **KEY POINT:** You can recognize the role a noun plays in a sentence through its case, and cases are marked by different endings to the stem.

3.2.1 Introduction to Cases: *a*-stem

> **KEY POINT:** Different categories of nouns change their form ("decline") differently. Nouns whose stems end in *-a* are very common and useful to learn.

This lesson is all about cases. Learning the cases is crucial for understanding Sanskrit sentences. But it's not easy. Take the noun योग (*yoga*) from our first lesson. This noun changes form depending on its case and number, as we learned in Lesson 2. Since there are eight cases and three different numbers, that's potentially twenty-four different forms of the noun to memorize. But that's not all—many nouns can be in the masculine, feminine, or neuter. So, multiply twenty-four times three. That's seventy-two. And then, there are different patterns depending on the spelling of the noun. Does it end with a vowel or a consonant? Which one? Arthur Anthony MacDonell's grammar has thirty-four pages of charts representing these patterns! Who could possibly remember so many thousands of variations? Don't fear. Two tools that can help the Sanskrit learner.

First, a handy tool for learning Sanskrit is called a *declension table* (these form changes are called *declensions*). As a Sanskrit student, my study space was full of declension tables, pasted on walls and doors. I recorded myself chanting them and listened to them as I jogged. This meant that when I came across a word in a sentence, I could (eventually) determine its grammatical gender, case, and number without consulting a dictionary. However, this is a lot of work. You can find the resources for this journey of memorization elsewhere.[1] We will be much more selective in this book. That's because of the other tool that helps us: patterns.

Below, we'll start with the declension table for the masculine noun योग (*yoga*) because it is a very common pattern. It's called the *a*-stem declension since it applies to nouns like योग (*yoga*) that end in अ (-*a*). I'm going to give you the whole chart twice—once in transliteration and once in Devanāgarī—please don't close the book even if it seems like a lot! Look them over, then read about how the cases work below. (Notice that some patterns repeat—these are in darker outlined boxes.) You can come back to the charts later. Once you start to see the patterns in declensions, learning new ones will be much easier since they tend to be variations on a theme. If you decide to take a course in Sanskrit, learning just a few of the declensions in this book will make your journey more manageable.

Table 12. *a*-stem masculine noun (*yoga*), transliteration only

	Singular	Dual	Plural
Nominative	yogaḥ	yogau	yogāḥ
Accusative	yogam	yogau	yogān
Instrumental	yogena	yogābhyām	yogaiḥ
Dative	yogāya	yogābhyām	yogebhyaḥ
Ablative	yogāt	yogābhyām	yogebhyaḥ
Genitive	yogasya	yogayoḥ	yogānām
Locative	yoge	yogayoḥ	yogeṣu
Vocative	yoga	yogau	yogāḥ

1. For example, you can use any of the textbooks listed in the Introduction to create flash cards on paper or in one of the many apps for language learning. Since these platforms will inevitably be outdated by the time of this book's publishing, I won't list them here, but a search for "flash card apps" will give you a lot to choose from.

Table 13. *a*-stem masculine noun (योग/*yoga*), Devanāgarī only

	Singular	Dual	Plural
Nominative	योगः	योगौ	योगाः
Accusative	योगम्	योगौ	योगान्
Instrumental	योगेन	योगाभ्याम्	योगैः
Dative	योगाय	योगाभ्याम्	योगेभ्यः
Ablative	योगात्	योगाभ्याम्	योगेभ्यः
Genitive	योगस्य	योगयोः	योगानाम्
Locative	योगे	योगयोः	योगेषु
Vocative	योग	योगौ	योगाः

Now that we've introduced the *a*-stem declension for masculine nouns, you can almost double your knowledge immediately by learning the *a*-stem declension for *neuter* nouns. It's identical, except for the first two cases (nominative and accusative). But the first two cases are the same in the neuter. For the rest, replace योग् (*yog-*) with वन् (*van-*), and you have the same pattern. Take a look, using वन (*vana*), which means "forest," as an example:

Table 14. *a*-stem neuter (*vana*), transliteration only

	Singular	Dual	Plural
Nominative	vanam	vane	vanāni
Accusative	vanam	vane	vanāni
Instrumental	vanena	vanābhyām	vanaiḥ
Dative	vanāya	vanābhyām	vanebhyaḥ
Ablative	vanāt	vanābhyām	vanebhyaḥ
Genitive	vanasya	vanayoḥ	vanānām
Locative	vane	vanayoḥ	vaneṣu
Vocative	vana	vane	vanāni

Table 15. *a*-stem neuter (वन/*vana*), Devanāgarī only

	Singular	Dual	Plural
Nominative	वनम्	वने	वनानि
Accusative	वनम्	वने	वनानि
Instrumental	वनेन	वनाभ्याम्	वनैः
Dative	वनाय	वनाभ्याम्	वनेभ्यः
Ablative	वनात्	वनाभ्याम्	वनेभ्यः
Genitive	वनस्य	वनयोः	वनानाम्
Locative	वने	वनयोः	वनेषु
Vocative	वन	वने	वनानि

3.2.2 Introduction to Cases: What They Do

KEY POINT: There are eight cases to know about in Sanskrit, many of which correspond to English prepositions.

To understand how cases work, let's step back and consider actions in general. Sentences are ways of expressing an action. Sometimes that action is pretty abstract, like *being* or *existing*. We've learned about the nominative already, which is the typical case for the subject of a sentence. In the example sentence from Lesson 2, योगश् चित्तवृत्तिनिरोधः (*yogaś cittavṛttinirodhaḥ*), the subject is योग (*yoga*). This sentence expresses what yoga is, which is why yoga is the subject. If we think about sentences as expressing actions, we can build Sanskrit sentences by combining subjects with actions.

The kind of sentence we'll focus on first is just one of four kinds of sentences we'll see in this book. The first two are when the subject is an agent, doing some action:

1. *Active transitive:* agent verbs object ("Rāma sees Sītā.")
2. *Passive transitive*: object is verbed by an agent ("Sītā is seen by Rāmā.")

The second two are when the subject is not an agent performing an action *on* some object. Instead, the verb expresses something about the subject itself, as we saw with yoga.

3. *Active intransitive*: subject verbs predicate ("Yoga is a discipline," "Rāma grew sorrowful.")
4. *Impersonal sentence*: subject verbs ("Yoga occurs," "Rāma sees.")

In what follows, we'll build an active, transitive sentence piece-by-piece, with Rāma as our agent, his name in the nominative case.[2]

2. Pandit point: Learning sentences with Rāma as the subject is now a bit of a trope in Sanskrit textbooks. While creative examples might be more fun, this approach allows us to learn some common vocabulary and use a name with a masculine declension. We'll learn sentences with grammatically feminine agents in the future.

Nominative case

The name "Rāma" is grammatically masculine and its ending is the same as योगः (*yogaḥ*), which makes it a simple example of the *nominative* case. For every word we add to the sentence, you can look back at the declension chart and see how its pattern matches the ending. The example follows a typical structure for Sanskrit sentences, but this order is pretty flexible because the cases give us lots of information.[3] We won't worry about applying sandhi in these examples, though I'll put it in the footnotes—these sentences have asterisks to remind you that they aren't what you'd see printed.

Pattern

<u>agent</u> verb

Example

*रामः गच्छति ।

<u>rāmaḥ</u> gacchati.[4]

<u>Rāma</u> travels.

We'll look at the verb in more detail below. For now, just know that *gacchati* is equivalent to *he/she/it travels*—it's the present tense in the singular third person. (Also notice that there are no capital letters in Devanāgarī, but when we translate names, we spell राम as "Rāma" not "rāma.")

3. Pandit point: How flexible is it? That's an area of investigation for linguists. An early paper on this is Staal (1967), developed by Gillon (1996). You can find discussion of both of these papers, along with discussion of Sanskrit grammarians on this topic, in Kulkarni, et al. (2013).

4. Pandit point: With sandhi, this sentence would be रामो गच्छति (*rāmo gacchati*). See Lesson 5. I am fairly certain I've heard stories of university Sanskrit students having shirts emblazoned with this sentence in homage to the constant use of Rāma's "going" as an example.

Accusative case

Let's have Rāma travel somewhere. The place he is going *to* is the object of his action. That means it would be in the *accusative*:

Pattern
agent object verb

Example
*रामः ग्रामम् गच्छति ।

rāmaḥ grāmam gacchati.[5]

Rāma travels to the village.

Notice that there are no prepositions like "to" in the Sanskrit sentence—the fact that we have an accusative singular ending lets us know that Rāma is going to a single village, not many villages. Likewise, there is no definite article "the" because that information is packed into the ending, -अम् (*-am*).

Instrumental case

Our third case is the *instrumental*, which expresses the means, the way that some agent performs an action.

Pattern
agent instrument object verb

Example
*रामः अश्वेन ग्रामम् गच्छति ।

rāmaḥ aśvena grāmam gacchati.[6]

Rāma travels to the village by horse.

---

5. Pandit point: With sandhi, this sentence would be रामो ग्रामं गच्छति (*rāmo grāmaṃ gacchati*). See Lesson 4 and Lesson 5.

6. Pandit point: With sandhi, this sentence would be रामो ऽश्वेन ग्रामं गच्छति (*rāmo 'śvena grāmaṃ gacchati*). See Lesson 4 and Lesson 5.

Again, the preposition "by" is unnecessary because the ending tells us that there is a single horse that Rāma is using as an instrument for his action—going. You'll notice that the English order doesn't match the Sanskrit order. It would sound strange to translate in Sanskrit order ("Rama by horse to the village travels"). Many Sanskrit students begin by translating this way, a kind of Yoda-Sanskrit. But it's better to translate it into natural-sounding English, even if this means reordering words.

If Rāma were doing fancy horse-riding—dressage—going astride two horses, we could convey that by saying:

Example

*रामः अश्वाभ्याम् ग्रामम् गच्छति ।

rāmaḥ aśvābhyām grāmam gacchati.[7]

Rāma travels to the village by two horses.

See if you can figure out how to say he travels by many horses. (An amazing feat that Rāma surely could accomplish!)

Dative case

Actions don't just happen, usually—they have a purpose. To express purpose, we use the *dative*:

Pattern

agent purpose instrument object verb

Example

*रामः धर्माय अश्वेन ग्रामम् गच्छति ।

rāmaḥ dharmāya aśvena grāmam gacchati.[8]

Rāma travels to the village by horse for a religious purpose.

---

7. Pandit point: With sandhi, this sentence would be रामो ऽश्वाभ्यां ग्रामं गच्छति (*rāmo 'śvābhyāṃ grāmaṃ gacchati*). See Lesson 4 and Lesson 5.

8. Pandit point: With sandhi, this sentence would be रामो धर्मायाश्वेन ग्रामं गच्छति (*rāmo dharmāyāśvena grāmaṃ gacchati*). See Lesson 4 and Lesson 5.

Yet again, we see that a preposition, here "for," is unnecessary in Sanskrit—the case ending informs us that there is a single purpose. While I've translated धर्म (*dharma*) so that we can compare English and Sanskrit sentences, that word is one of many that resists easy translation. (Also, see 3.2.4 below for the *r* in *dharma*—it's the little curl at the top.) Depending on the context, *dharma* can mean rule, virtue, righteousness, religion, devotion, or even—in certain Buddhist philosophical uses—the fundamental components of reality. Lesson 13 talks more about translation challenges.

Ablative case

There are three more cases we can add to our ever-expanding sentence. The *ablative* expresses the action's being *apart from* something. Rāma travels *to* the village, but he is leaving *from* somewhere. Let's imagine he's traveling from the ocean—that is his origin point:

Pattern

agent purpose instrument origin object verb

Example

*रामः धर्माय अश्वेन सागरात् ग्रामम् गच्छति ।

rāmaḥ dharmāya aśvena sāgarāt grāmam gacchati.[9]

Rāma travels from the ocean to the village by horse for a religious purpose.

9. Pandit point: With sandhi, this sentence would be रामो धर्मायाश्वेन सागराद्ग्रामं गच्छति (*rāmo dharmāyāśvena sāgarādgrāmaṃ gacchati*). You might have to squint to see that there's a consonant conjunct of three consonants, *-dgr*, which is unusual but can happen. Here's a bigger version: द्ग्र (*-dgr*), and you can see Lesson 4, Lesson 5, and Lesson 7 for sandhi.

Genitive case

The *genitive* case[10] is a hard-working, all-purpose kind of case that expresses a relationship, like owning or belonging. Usually the genitive goes before the noun that it modifies. It's anachronistic, but let's imagine Rāma is going to visit the Buddha in his village. We can express this with the genitive, the "village *of* the Buddha," or just "the Buddha's village," बुद्धस्य ग्रामम् (*buddhasya grāmam*):

Pattern

agent purpose instrument origin <u>owner</u> object verb

Example

*रामः धर्माय अश्वेन सागरात् बुद्धस्य ग्रामम् गच्छति ।

rāmaḥ dharmāya aśvena sāgarāt <u>buddhasya</u> grāmam gacchati.[11]

Rāma travels from the ocean to <u>the Buddha's</u> village (the village <u>of the Buddha</u>) by horse for a religious purpose.

---

10. Pandit point: Sanskrit grammarians like Pāṇini might be very upset with me at this point. The genitive isn't strictly a case for them—or at least, not if we identify the Sanskrit term *kāraka* with case. There are six *kārakas*: *apādāna* (fixed origin), *sampradāna* (aim), *karaṇa* (instrument), *adhikaraṇa* (location), *karman* (object), and *kartṛ* (agent). These correspond to (in order) ablative, dative, instrumental, locative, accusative, and nominative cases. On this understanding, *kārakas* express the relationships between verbs and nouns. But genitives (and vocatives, see below) express the relationship between two nouns. You can read about this issue elsewhere: the relationship between case and Sanskrit grammatical concepts, especially the subject/nominative, is complex. But see Cardona (1974) and Gillon (2007).

11. Pandit point: With sandhi, this sentence would be रामो धर्मायाश्वेन सागराद्बुद्धस्य ग्रामं गच्छति (*rāmo dharmāyāśvena sāgarādbuddhasya grāmaṃ gacchati*). Another new conjunct, with a vowel added, to boot. Here's a bigger version: द्बु (*-dbu*), and you can see Lesson 4, Lesson 5, and Lesson 7 for sandhi.

Locative case

Our seventh case, the *locative*, does what its name suggests. It gives the *location* of an action. Where is Rāma doing the action of going? He is traveling in a kingdom, so we add our locative singular ending:

Pattern

agent location purpose instrument origin owner object verb

Example

*रामः राज्ये धर्माय अश्वेन सागरात् बुद्धस्य ग्रामम् गच्छति ।

rāmaḥ rājye dharmāya aśvena sāgarāt buddhasya grāmam gacchati.[12]

Rāma travels in the kingdom from the ocean to the Buddha's village by horse for a religious purpose.

Vocative case

Phew! We could make this sentence more complex, but let's stop with one last case, the vocative. The *vocative* is a way of addressing someone. So, if I were to address this sentence to you, the reader, I might say:

Pattern

addressee! agent location purpose instrument origin owner object verb

Example

*शिष्य रामः राज्ये धर्माय अश्वेन सागरात् बुद्धस्य ग्रामम् गच्छति ।

śiṣya rāmaḥ rājye dharmāya aśvena sāgarāt buddhasya grāmam gacchati.[13]

---

12. Pandit point: With sandhi, this sentence would be रामो राज्ये धर्मायाश्वेन सागराद्बुद्धस्य ग्रामं गच्छति (*rāmo rājye dharmāyāśvena sāgarādbuddhasya grāmaṃ gacchati*).

13. Pandit point: No new sandhi for this sentence. But, like the genitive, the vocative isn't what most Sanskrit grammarians consider a case (or a close equivalent to the case, the *kāraka*).

Student! Rāma travels in the kingdom from the ocean to the Buddha's village by horse for a religious purpose.

We can use these cases in other ways, and we'll encounter some of them as we read. They can have extended senses, which are not so physical as the example sentence. The ablative case ("from") can refer to a physical origin, but it can also refer to an abstract origin—the basis for our thinking, a reason. ("From *this*, I conclude *that*.") For now, if you want to try out your new knowledge, consider how you might replace the singular forms of the nouns above with dual or plural ones based on the patterns in the declension chart. Notice that some cases overlap in form, meaning you will need to watch out and pay attention to context when reading.

3.2.3 Verbs: Introduction to 1P and Thematic Verbs

KEY POINT: Sanskrit verbs are formed by adding endings onto a verb stem. Knowing what class a verb is in helps us recognize the patterns that create this stem.

At last, we come to our first verb. You might be thinking, "Finally! What can we do without verbs?!" But remember that nominal sentences, which we introduced earlier, are very common in Sanskrit. In fact, depending on the genre, you may not encounter many verbs but mostly read nominal sentences and compounds. Still, verbs are helpful because they allow us to locate our words in time—we can talk about things in the past, present, and future, as well as order people to do things and talk about what might have been.

Notation

Let's start by understanding the notation in our vocabulary list. I've written the verb भू (*bhū*) with a square root symbol in front, √, which might be surprising in a book about language. Don't worry. I'm not asking you to take the square root of a word! This is just a standard way to mark that the word is a verb *root*. Verb roots are the fundamental parts of the verb, on which we make changes depending on things like tense and number. The verb root √*bhū* is thus something like the word "be," which we find in an English dictionary entry. It's how you look up the verb in a Sanskrit dictionary. Similar to √*bhū*, English speakers transform "be" into a range of forms, depending on tense ("I *was*," "I *am*," "I *will be*") and number ("I *am*," "They *are*"). The difference is that, unlike "be," which can appear in a sentence ("She will *be* there"), in Sanskrit, you will never see the root form √*bhū* used as the main verb in a sentence.

Beside the verb, in parentheses, are a number and letter: 1P. You'll see this label in a dictionary, and it will provide you with useful information. The number tells you what the class of the verb is, and the letter tells you it is in active voice (we will wait for Lesson 10 to get deeper into this distinction).[14] To see how this information helps us, compare √भू (*bhū*) to the English word "be." That verb changes in some strange ways—it starts with the letter "b" in the dictionary, but when you *conjugate* it (change it depending on tense, voice, and mood), sometimes it starts with "w," other times with "a," and sometimes you add an entirely new word before it! Sanskrit verbs conjugate according to ten regular patterns, in contrast. If you know a verb's class (1 through 10) and voice, you know what pattern it follows when conjugating.

Verb classes

KEY POINT: A verb root is marked with two pieces of information in a dictionary: the class (1–10) and the voice (P, A). These tell you about the pattern it follows.

14. Pandit point: the "P" stands for a Sanskrit word, *parasmaipada* (परस्मैपद), which tells us it is probably a transitive verb. *Parasmaipada* is a compound, literally "a word (*pada*) that is for something else (*parasmai*)." This compound is different from the ones we've learned about so far since it includes the dative case ending for पर (*para*).

Our verb root √*bhū* is part of the first class, and that lets us look it up in any number of grammar books to see what pattern it follows. What's nice about learning this verb is that its conjugation pattern is very similar to several other classes, known as *thematic* classes. These include 1, 4, 6, and 10. By learning how √भू (*bhū*) conjugates, you'll have a sense of how these other verbs work.

Now, strictly speaking, there are verb roots and verb stems.[15] The root first takes some changes to become a stem, and then endings designating person and number are added. A plant metaphor can help you: The verbal root is the unseen starting point from which a verb grows into a stem. Onto the stem are added other components (like leaves and flowers). The stem of √भू (*bhū*) is भव (*bhava*). The reason has to do with some sandhi we'll learn later in Lesson 6.[16] Knowing which class a verb root belongs to will help you learn the patterns that produce its stem shown in Table 16 and Table 17.

The letter "P" tells us this verb is in the *active* voice, and it tells us that there's a specific pattern the verb should follow. Verbs marked with an "A" are *middle* voice, and they follow a different pattern.[17] Sometimes the same verb root can follow either pattern. In a dictionary, the information in parentheses tells you which pattern(s) the verb follows. In this book, the notation tells you which form is being used in a chapter, even if it can conjugate in both. Here, the verb root √भू (*bhū*) follows the 1P pattern.

15. Pandit point: For some verbs, the root and the stem are the same (it's a *root stem*). This is the case for another important verb meaning "to be," √अस् (*as*), which we'll encounter in Lesson 4.

16. Pandit point: The quick explanation is that a strengthening process (*guṇa*), which we learn about in Lesson 6, transforms the verbal root √भू (*bhū*) into भो (*bho*). Then, the vowel अ (*a*) is added to the stem. The vowel ओ (*o*) in contact with अ (*a*) becomes a semi-vowel, व (*va*), through sandhi we also learn in Lesson 6. This results in भव (*bhava*), which takes the ending -ति (*-ti*).

17. Pandit point: "A" is for ātmanepada (आत्मनेपद), "a word (*pada*) that is for itself (*ātmane*)."

These "P" verbs are often *transitive*, meaning they typically take objects, like:

1. The queen *slays* the lion.
2. The bird *eats* the food.
3. The student *reads* the book.

You might notice that some of these sentences, (2) and (3), could be written without the objects (the food, the book).[18] If we do that, the verb becomes *intransitive*—there's no object needed, and we're focusing on how the action impacts the person (or animal) doing it—the effect on the agent. The "A" and "P," or *active* and *middle* distinction, isn't the same as the difference between transitive and intransitive, though it may have been long ago. With this in mind, look at the pattern of endings in Table 16 and Table 17 for the present tense, or actions occurring right now (the present indicative).

Table 16. Present indicative verb endings, 1P

	Singular (one)	Dual (two)	Plural (more than two)
Third person (he/she/they)	-ति (-ti)	-तः (-taḥ)	-अन्ति (-anti)
Second person (you)	-सि (-si)	-थः (-thaḥ)	-थ (-tha)
First person (I)	-मि (-mi)	-वः (-vaḥ)	-मः (-maḥ)

These endings are added to our verb stem, *bhava*, which results in the pattern below:

18. In contemporary slang, we could even rewrite the first one as intransitive: "The queen slays" could be used when talking about how Beyonce's attire at a music awards event was beautiful and well-chosen.

Table 17. Present indicative √भू (*bhū*) (1P) - to be, to exist

	Singular	Dual	Plural
Third person	भवति (bhava**ti**) - he/she/it is	भवतः (bhava**taḥ**) - those two are	भवन्ति (bhava**nti**) - they are
Second person	भवसि (bhava**si**) - you are	भवथः (bhava**thaḥ**) - you two are	भवथ (bhava**tha**) - you all are
First person	भवामि (bhavā**mi**) - I am	भवावः (bhavā**vaḥ**) - we two are	भवामः (bhavā**maḥ**) - we are

You might notice that the first person भव + मि (*bhava* + *mi*) results in भवामि (*bhavāmi*). The long *ā* in this form and the first person dual and plural results from the short *a* lengthening to a long *ā*.

3.2.4 The *Repha*

There's a new quirk of Devanāgarī to explain before you read this text, and that has to do with one of the symbols which has a name, the रेफ (*repha*):

र्

Sometimes, it creeps on top of the long horizontal line (called the *headline*). This has happened in the word दर्शन (*darśana*) in our reading when the *repha* encountered a consonant:

दर् + शन

dar + śana

The *repha* will become a smaller, curled symbol that then appears above the next sound to be pronounced. Here, that's the श (*śa*):

दर्श

darśa

The complete word is therefore printed:

दर्शन

darśana

Since the next sound to be pronounced is श (*śa*), the *repha* appears above श, whose symbol implicitly includes the *a* sound. But if the next sound to be pronounced were शा (*śā*), the *repha* would appear above the combination of the *ś* and the long *ā*, printed as शा below:

दर्शा

darśā

This is why we see the dative singular form, *dharmāya*, as धर्माय in the examples above. Now, if the *repha* encounters a consonant conjunct, it will appear at the end of the conjunct. Here's an extreme example:

कार् + त्स्न्य

kār + tsnya

कार्त्स्न्य

kārtsnya

Understanding this pattern is important for reading Devanāgarī since so many common words have the *repha* in this position. For example, see if you can read and transliterate what would be the first line of a declension table for the masculine *a*-stem अर्थ, below (answer at the end of the lesson):

अर्थः अर्थौ अर्थाः

3.3 Putting Everything Together

धूमप्रत्यक्षदर्शनात् अग्नौ अनुमानम् भवति ।

dhūmapratyakṣadarśanāt agnau anumānam bhavati.[19]

19. I have simplified sandhi in this reading so as not to introduce too much too quickly. See Lesson 7 for an explanation of what would happen to the -त् (*-t*) when it encounters अ- (*a-*), Lesson 6 for what would happen to the final diphthong in अग्नौ (*agnau*) before अ- (*a-*), and Lesson 4 for -म् (*-m*) when it encounters भ- (*bh-*).

In our reading, we have a main verb at the end of an intransitive sentence, भवति (*bhavati*). It matches the subject of our sentence, अनुमानम् (*anumānam*), in number (check your tables to see if it is singular, dual, or plural). While the form of the nominative and accusative are the same for the neuter *a*-stem, because there is no other candidate noun for the subject, it seems likely to be the subject, so nominative. These two words express the main action of the sentence, अनुमानम् भवति (*anumānam bhavati*), since there is no other candidate noun in the nominative to make this a sentence saying what *anumāna* is, like when we say "A tree is an oak."

> धूमप्रत्यक्षदर्शनात् अग्नौ **अनुमानम् भवति ।**
> *dhūmapratyakṣadarśanāt agnau* **inference occurs/exists.**

The other two words in the sentence tell us more about inference. The first word in the sentence is a compound made up of three words. Its head noun (see 2.2.4) is in the ablative case, -दर्शनात् (*-darśanāt*). This case expresses the idea of coming from some fixed position or, more abstractly, an event or process that comes from some starting place:

> **धूमप्रत्यक्षदर्शनात्** अग्नौ अनुमानम् भवति ।
> **from-*dhūmapratyakṣadarśana*** *agnau* inference occurs/exists.
>
> **because of-*dhūmapratyakṣadarśana*** *agnau* inference occurs/exists.

The second word follows a different declension pattern than the *a*-stem we've learned in this chapter, but it is a locative singular noun. Its stem form is अग्नि (*agni*), so that's how I've spelled it in the gloss below. As with our other cases, the locative can have different meanings. Sometimes, it means "on" or "in," but it can also be a *locative of topic*, which expresses what something is about:

धूमप्रत्यक्षदर्शनात् अग्नौ अनुमानम् भवति ।

from/because of-*dhūmapratyakṣadarśana* **in *agni*** inference occurs/exists.

from/because of-*dhūmapratyakṣadarśana* **about *agni*** inference occurs/exists.

Now, see if you can interpret the compound using your vocabulary list and what you learned in Lesson 2. You will almost certainly want to reorder the words into natural-sounding English. The core of the sentence is that inference—a kind of reasoning—exists or occurs under certain conditions. (Read on for some hints about what the sentence means.)

3.4 About the Reading: Where There's Smoke, There's Fire

Philosophy in the Indian subcontinent was much more than just Yoga. This lesson's reading is written by a thinker from the tradition known as Nyāya (न्याय in Devanāgarī, notice the initial consonant conjunct).[20] While Nyāya philosophers probably followed some yogic practices, they take a different text than the *Yogasūtra* as their starting point. This text is called, appropriately, the *Nyāyasūtra*, or loosely, *Aphorisms on Right Reason*. The *Nyāyasūtra* was collected by Vātsyāyana, the author of the *Nyāyabhāṣya*, our reading for this lesson. The *sūtra*'s systematic collection of statements was transmitted orally for a long time

20. Pandit point: The initial न्य (*ny*-) of Nyāya can be difficult for English speakers to pronounce. It should be pronounced like the *ny* in "ca**ny**on" without any intervening vowel. (If you are a fan of the Three Stooges—Larry, Curly, and Moe—think of saying "**ny**uk **ny**uk **ny**uk." Be aware this is only an approximation since Larry's pronunciation of "ny" is a palatal nasal, like ञ् (*ñ*). But it might help you avoid inserting an extra vowel!)

until Vātsyāyana, around 450 CE, put it together, along with his commentary (*bhāṣya*).[21]

One of the main topics of Nyāya was knowledge, and these philosophers identified four main ways we can come to know truth. Two of these make an appearance in our reading: perception and inference. In this excerpt, Vātsyāyana is explaining *Nyāyasūtra* 2.1.32, which is about the relationship between these two ways of knowing. Inference and perception are not the same. Perception is a way of knowing that results from our senses, like eyesight, coming into contact with objects. But inference is a further step. It starts with a perceptual experience, like seeing smoke (*dhūma*) on a distant mountain. However, Nyāya philosophers argue that inference brings together this perception with our memory of a regularity: whenever there is smoke, there is fire (*agni*). And since there's smoke on that distant mountain, because of this rule, we know that there is fire on that distant mountain and can draw an inference about that fire. A deceptively simple idea, inference is subject to many further characterizations in Nyāya thought, which allows these philosophers to analyze its structure and distinguish good from bad reasoning.

Self-Quiz Answers

*रामः अश्वैः ग्रामम् गच्छति ।
rāmaḥ <u>aśvaiḥ</u> grāmam gacchati.[22]
Rāma travels to the village <u>by many horses</u>.
अर्थः (*arthaḥ*) अर्थौ (*arthau*) अर्थाः (*arthāḥ*)
This is the word for "meaning" or "purpose," which we'll see in Lesson 7.

---

21. See Lesson 12 for a discussion of commentary in Sanskrit. Commentaries exist for a range of genres: philosophy, literature, grammar, ritual, astrology, medicine, and more. For a guide to the *Nyāyabhāṣya*, see Dasti (2023).

22. Pandit point: With sandhi, this sentence would be रामो ऽश्वैर्ग्रामं गच्छति (*rāmo 'śvair grāmaṃ gacchati*). We don't discuss this sandhi change in this guide, but it has to do with encountering voiced consonants, which we do talk about in Lesson 5.

Lesson 4

Reading: Bṛhadāraṇyaka Upaniṣad 1.4.10

अहं ब्रह्मास्मि ।

ahaṃ brahmāsmi.

Points of Interest For

The Curious: You can focus on the verb in 4.2.3 and the nominative singular form of the pronoun to understand the reading.

The Yoga Aficionado: If you are familiar with Vedānta already, read about two important Vedānta philosophers in 4.3 About the Reading.

The Scholar: You can compare the 2P verb in this lesson with the 1P in Lesson 3 to appreciate their shared patterns.

4.1 Vocabulary

Devanāgarī	Transliteration	Part of Speech	Translation
अक्षर	akṣara	neut. n.	a syllable; the syllable *oṃ*
√अस्	√as	v. (2P)	to be, to exist
अस्मद्	asmad	1 pn.	I/we
आरण्यक	āraṇyaka	neut. n.	name for a type of text recited in a forest
उपनिषद्	upaniṣad	fem. n.	name for texts that contain teachings about the self, existence, ritual
बृहत्[1]	bṛhat	adj.	great
ब्रह्म	brahma	n., neut. nom. sg. form of ब्रह्मन् (brahman)	the Absolute, the divine; truth; the Vedas
ं	ṃ (the *anusvāra*)	a symbol for nasal consonant	
वाक्य	vākya	neut. n.	sentence

1. To understand why this word changes to बृहद् (*bṛhad*) in the title of this lesson's reading, look at Lesson 7.

4.2 Grammar Notes

KEY POINT: Different categories of verbs change (conjugate) differently. In this lesson, we'll see how 2P verbs differ from 1P verbs we learned in Lesson 3.

This lesson's sentence, which consists of three words, is known as one of the "Great Sentences" in one of the most famous and oldest Sanskrit texts in world literature: the *Upaniṣads*.[2] This particular Great (*mahā-*) Sentence (*vākya*) packs a lot of philosophical ideas into just three words, and philosophers worldwide have written volumes on understanding them. There's even a "Vedic metal" band in Singapore named Rudra, which uses these sentences in their lyrics![3] Long ago, when Vedic metal would have meant copper and iron, the text that we're reading was composed (or revealed, depending on your view) and transmitted orally for generations. This was probably sometime in the sixth to seventh century BCE, but, as with most of these ancient texts, dating is tricky. The *Great "Āraṇyaka" Upaniṣad* includes dialogues, debates, and stories, and it reflects on the relationship between ancient rituals and the structure of the universe. Its name resists easy translation since आरण्यक (*āraṇyaka*) means "related to the forest," a type of text that was recited (and maybe composed) in the forest wilderness away from civilization.[4]

---

2. Pandit point: Since the plural for the Sanskrit उपनिषद् (*upaniṣad*) is not formed by adding an "-s" to the end, I do not italicize the final "-s." This is a typographic convention that many, but not all, writers follow when making an English plural out of a Sanskrit term. You might want to know how to make its plural in Sanskrit. Well, that depends on the case, as we've seen. Its nominative plural form is उपनिषदः (*upaniṣadaḥ*). In the nominative singular, it is spelled उपनिषत् (*upaniṣat*). You can look up the full declension in a grammar book.

3. The sentence is the title of a song and also appears in the song from their album *Brahmavidya: Primordial I*. Dairianathan (2012) discusses their work in some detail, for the curious.

4. In brief, an *Āraṇyaka* is a kind of text that inquires into deeper meanings of ritual actions described in other texts, not unlike what the *Upaniṣads* do. And the *Bṛhadāraṇyaka*

Among other questions, it asks: How did the world come about? What's the relationship between our selves and ultimate reality? All this is packed into this text—and these three words. To understand, we need to start with a little more sandhi.

4.2.1 Vowel Sandhi: Similar Vowel Combinations

> **KEY POINT:** Any two similar simple vowels in combination, like *a* + *ā* or *ī* + *ī*, result in a long vowel, like *ā* or *ī*.

We have already seen that sound changes are represented in Devanāgarī, so when words come together, their forms sometimes change. In Lesson 2, we focused on consonants. Not only do consonants change when they come into contact with each other, but vowels do, too. The first main distinction we need to make is whether the vowels that come into contact are similar or dissimilar. If they're similar, the simple vowels, whether long or short, will lengthen into a long vowel, as shown in Table 18. (The diphthongs and the semi-vocalic ṛ have different rules. A *diphthong* is a single vowel sound made from two vowels combined, like "ou" in "hour," in contrast to the "oo" in "cooperate," which remains two sounds.) Here's the pattern for similar vowels. I'll represent all of them with अ (*a*) and आ (*ā*), but the pattern is the same for all the others: they combine into the long vowel.

Upaniṣad holds a kind of in-between status, both *Āraṇyaka* and *Upaniṣad*. Olivelle (2008) explains these genres of text in more detail in the introduction to his translation of the *Upaniṣads*, xxx–xxxiii.

Table 18. Vowel sandhi, similar vowel combinations

First Vowel	Second Vowel		Combination	Example
अ (*a*)	अ (*a*)		आ (*ā*)	dhūma agni → dhūmāgni धूम अग्नि → धूमाग्नि
अ (*a*)	आ (*ā*)	→	आ (*ā*)	yoga āsana → yogāsana योग आसन→ योगासन
आ (*ā*)	अ (*a*)		आ (*ā*)	brahmā akṣara- → brahmākṣara ब्रह्मा अक्षर → ब्रह्माक्षर
आ (*ā*)	आ (*ā*)		आ (*ā*)	brahmā āsana- → brahmāsana ब्रह्मा आसन→ ब्रह्मासन

However, the situation with dissimilar vowels is more complex. We'll talk about why in Lesson 6.

4.2.2 Nasal Sandhi: *Anusvāra*

KEY POINT: If you see the after-sound ◌ं, you can break sandhi and replace it with म्.

In this section, you're going to learn one more letter, the अनुस्वार (*anusvāra*)—it looks like a small dot, and we see it in our reading.[5] It's a result of sandhi, and the transliterated form is easy to remember since it also includes a small dot: *ṃ*

अहं (*ahaṃ*)

To understand the sandhi that results in this letter, quickly say the following pairs of words out loud:

ten ten keys
ten ten bucks

5. Pandit point: The term अनुस्वार (*anusvāra*) means "after-sound."

If you pay attention, you'll notice that on its own, the "n" in "ten" is pronounced more strongly, but when "keys" or "bucks" follow, the "n" sound changes slightly. That "n" is a nasal consonant. The sound changes in anticipation of the upcoming consonant. By now, you will recognize the implication for Sanskrit—when this change happens, we spell the words differently.

The symbol for the nasal consonant looks like a little dot. It appears just above the horizontal line—the headline—that we talked about in the Introduction, like below.

कं (*kaṃ*) or किं (*kiṃ*)

This consonant is pronounced like "m," although it slightly borrows the sound of the consonant that comes after it, as does the "n" in "ten bucks" and "ten keys." When do we see this dot appear? We can think of it as a replacement for -म् (*-m*) when that consonant, at the end of a word, bumps up against another consonant. It'd be like changing the "n" at the end of "ten" to show how it sounds when we say "ten bucks." But -म् (*-m*) doesn't change when it comes into contact with a vowel.[6]

Table 19. Nasal sandhi, *anusvāra*

Final Sound	Initial Sound		Combination	Example
म् (*m*)	consonant	→	◌ं + consonant	sūtram nirodhaḥ → sūtraṃ nirodhaḥ सूत्रम् निरोधः → सूत्रं निरोधः
म् (*m*)	vowel		_म् + vowel	vākyam akṣaram = vākyam akṣaram वाक्यम् अक्षरम् = वाक्यम् अक्षरम्

6. Pandit point: The principles of sandhi around nasals are more complex than this, and there are five different nasals into which म् (*m*) can transform when it comes into contact with consonants. In this book, we'll use the *anusvāra* for all of these cases.

4.2.3 Verbs: Introduction to 2P and Athematic Verbs

> **KEY POINT:** 2P verbs have a different pattern in the singular than the dual conjugation.

In the last lesson, we learned the 1P verb √भू (*bhū*). In this lesson, we'll look at the 2P verb √अस् (*as*), which is second class, *parasmaipada*. 1P verbs are *thematic* verbs—they share very similar patterns with 4, 6, and 10. In contrast, 2P is *athematic*. The only thing athematic verbs have in common is that they differ from thematic verbs. Each athematic class (2, 3, 5, 7, 8, and 9) has a slightly different conjugation pattern.

In the second class, there is something unusual happening, known as a *root stem*. Although we saw that the root √भू (*bhū*) "grows" into the stem भव (*bhava*), the second class stem is the same as its root, just as we see in our example verb: √अस् (*as*). This means our endings, like ति (*ti*), go directly onto the root stem: अस्ति (*asti*), as in Table 20. Another unusual change in this verb is that its initial अ (*a*) basically disappears in six of the forms (the dual and plural), leaving just स् (*s*) for the endings. Not all verbs in the second class are like this. But they are like √अस् (*as*) in having some different patterns in the singular compared to the dual and plural.[7] Irregularities like this tend to happen with frequently used words—like people, popular words can be weird without much issue, while the rest conform closely to the standard patterns.

7. Pandit point: The difference is between the strong and weak forms. In the present indicative, the singular forms are strong, and the dual and plural forms are weak. We'll return to the idea of strengthening later in Lesson 6.

Table 20. Present indicative √अस् (*as*) (2P) - to be, to exist

	Singular	Dual	Plural
Third person	अस्ति (asti) - he/she/it is	स्तः (staḥ) - those two are	सन्ति (santi) - they are
Second person	असि (asi) - you are	स्थः (sthaḥ) - you two are	स्थ (stha) - you all are
First person	अस्मि (asmi) - I am	स्वः (svaḥ) - we two are	स्मः (smaḥ) - we are

Before we move on, look at the table and see if you can identify any of these forms of √अस् (*as*) in the reading. A hint is to look for the endings and check for any potential sandhi that might have impacted the vowels.

4.2.4 Personal Pronouns: First Person

KEY POINT: First-personal pronouns in Sanskrit decline, just like nouns decline.

The last part of speech we'll introduce is the first personal pronoun—the word for "I" or "we." As with the nouns we discussed in the last lesson, pronouns change form depending on whether they're referring to the subject or object and how many subjects or objects there are. Although the king of England may use "we," most people, when one person is speaking, will say, "*I* am reading a book." In contrast, if talking about yourself and some friends, you would say, "*We* are playing lacrosse." By now, you know that Sanskrit has a dual number, so you could easily say, "*We two* are playing ping pong" just by changing the pronoun "we" (in Sanskrit) to have a different ending. For now, let's stick to the nominative, which is the form we use when the pronoun is the subject of a sentence.

Table 21. First-personal pronoun, अस्मद् (*asmad*)

	Singular	Dual	Plural
Nominative (subject)	अहम् (aham) - I	आवाम् (āvām) - we two	वयम् (vayam) - we

With these pronouns and the first-person forms of the verb √अस् (*as*), we can now make three basic sentences. Below is one example with sandhi. See if you can construct the other two.

आवां स्वः (*avaṃ svaḥ*)

We two are.

As a reminder from Lesson 3, the Sanskrit verb typically goes at the end, like this:

Pattern

noun1 noun2 verb = the noun1 verbs noun2

Another way to put this is:

Pattern

subject object verb = the subject verbs the object[8]

We can also identify another pattern:

subject predicate is-verb = the subject *is* the predicate.

A *predicate* gives information about the subject, while the *object* takes the action of the verb. In Lesson 2, we saw subjects (like "yoga") identified with predicates (like "cessation") in nominal sentences without a verb ("yoga is the cessation"). You can now make nominal sentences with the verb √अस् (*as*) or √भू (*bhū*). You only need to make sure the predicate matches the verb in number (and person, when it's a pronoun).

8. See Lesson 5 for further refinement: transitive verbs take objects, while intransitive verbs do not.

Whether the predicate is a noun or a pronoun, it must match the verb, as in the underlined portion below:

> **Example**
> *<u>वनं</u> राज्यम् <u>अस्ति</u> (<u>vanaṃ</u> *rājyam* <u>asti</u>)[9]
>
> <u>The forest is</u> the kingdom.

In this sentence, the two things—the forest and the kingdom—are being equated. Notice that the predicate is singular, and the verb is also singular. Because the subject is a thing (the forest), the verb is in the third person. Imagine a subject proudly addressing their ruler and hyperbolically saying:

> **Example**
> *<u>अहं</u> राज्यम् <u>अस्मि</u> (<u>ahaṃ</u> *rājyam* <u>asmi</u>)[10]
>
> <u>I am</u> the kingdom.

Here, even though राज्यम् (*rājyam*) is singular, it cannot be the subject because the verb is in the first-person singular. The subject must be अहम् (*aham*). (Even if the pronoun wasn't there, we could know this by the verb's conjugation.)

4.3 Putting Everything Together

> अहं ब्रह्मास्मि ।
>
> ahaṃ brahmāsmi.

In your vocabulary list, you have the word ब्रह्म (*brahma*), which is in the neuter nominative singular form, just like we saw योगः (*yogaḥ*) last

9. In printed Devanāgarī, this would read राज्यमस्ति. See 6.2.3, for why.

10. In printed Devanāgarī, this would also read differently. See if you can guess based on the previous footnote.

lesson and have now learned अहम् (*aham*) this lesson. Their endings are all different, but they are all in the nominative.

With this in mind, go back and read the Great Sentence above. First, as always, check for places where sandhi might change the spelling of words: there is an *anusvāra* in the sentence as well as a long vowel. Second, look for a verb and determine its person (first, second, or third) and number (singular, dual, or plural). See if any of the words in the sentence match the person and number of the verb. Remember the subject–object–verb pattern, and see if you can understand this Great (three-word) Sentence.

4.4 About the Reading: Ways of Being Brahman

What does it mean to equate myself with Brahman? And what does the word "Brahman" mean in the first place? These are questions that people have been asking for thousands of years. Our lesson's sentence appears in the *Great Āraṇyaka Upaniṣad*, in a section that describes the creation of everything. (There are lots of creation stories in the *Upaniṣads*; this is just one of them.) The only existing thing, Brahman, thinks this sentence about itself. It then "becomes the whole world."[11] Each kind of thing that comes to exist—gods and human beings—thinks this sentence and also "becomes the whole world."

Because the word ब्रह्मन् (*brahman*) seems to refer to something that thinks and acts, it's often written with a capital letter as a proper name: "Brahman." But it isn't just a god. It comes before the gods and is often described as the cause of everything that exists. And sometimes, it's identified as being the same thing as our individual selves. What that means is something that philosophers like Śaṅkara and Rāmānuja discuss hundreds of years after the *Upaniṣads*. Śaṅkara argues that there's

11. Olivelle (2008, 15); Dairianathan (2012).

just one thing that exists—Brahman—and everything else is an illusion. Rāmānuja argues that Brahman is the most fundamental thing that exists—and all other things exist in dependence on Brahman. In a sense, they are ways that Brahman exists. These philosophers were not part of the Yoga tradition discussed in Lesson 2, but another tradition known as Vedānta.[12]

One last point: Remember the word नमस्ते (*namaste*), which we discussed in the introduction and Lesson 2? Although it is used to mean "hello!" as a very ordinary greeting, some people—both modern yoga practitioners and premodern South Asian thinkers—argue that the term can have a further meaning in some contexts. You may have heard it: "The divine in me bows to the divine in you." If everyone is Brahman in some sense, then even though ते (*te*) is just an ordinary personal pronoun, in a dative form that means "for/to you," before the beginning of a yoga session, saying नमस्ते (*namaste*) suggests honoring the divine which is identified as your self.[13] This goes beyond the dictionary meaning of the words, though. If you were to say to the king of England, "It's an honor to meet you," your words might suggest something weightier about the *honor* and *you* than if you say the same thing to a nonroyal new acquaintance.

12. Pandit point: You can use your knowledge of Sanskrit compounds and vowel sandhi to understand this word. Vedānta (वेदान्त) means the "end" (*anta*) of the Veda (*veda*). The Veda is a set of ancient, orally transmitted texts that include hymns, myths, and poetry—and the *Upaniṣads* are not just after them (at their "end" chronologically), but Vedānta philosophers think they are also their whole point, the "end" in the sense of their aim.

13. Pandit point: Phillips suggests this (2009, 272n26), and Indian thinkers like Vedānta Deśika also provide analyses of the word that give it several layers of meaning. This shortened dative form, an *enclitic*, is printed in Appendix 1 (we won't learn it in a lesson).

Lesson 5

Reading: Kāmasūtra 1.2.30

न निष्कर्मणो भद्रम् अस्तीति
वात्स्यायनः।

na niṣkarmaṇo bhadram astīti vātsyāyanaḥ.

Points of Interest For

The Curious: Focus on reading about genitives in 5.2.2 and exocentric compounds in 5.2.5.

The Yoga Aficionado: Watch out for why निर्वाण (*nirvāṇa*) has the form it does.

The Scholar: Look at the voiced and unvoiced patterns in Table 22 and then revisit Lesson 3.

5.1 Vocabulary

Devanāgarī	Transliteration	Part of Speech	Translation
इति	iti	indc.	"" (quotation marker)
कर्मन्	karman	neut. n.	action, activity, effort
काम	kāma	masc. n	desire, love
न	na	ind.	no (negation of verb)
निष्-	niṣ-	pfx. (from *nis*)	without, non-
प्रयोजन	prayojana	neut n.	purpose, goal
भद्र	bhadra	neut. n.	prosperity, good fortune
वात्स्यायन	vātsyāyana	masc. n., proper name	Vātsyāyana
बहु	bahu	adj.	many, much, a lot
व्रीहि	vrīhi	masc. n.	rice
निर्वाण	nirvāṇa	neut. n.	blowing out, extinction

5.2 Grammar Notes

KEY POINTS: Compounds are a compressed way of expressing the relationships among different words without using case endings. However, understanding cases is important for understanding compounds.

Perhaps you're wondering why a reputable publisher like Hackett let one of its authors excerpt the *Kāmasūtra* in a book about learning Sanskrit. In the popular imagination, the *Kāmasūtra* is a very "adult" text, even mildly scandalous. While it's true that it has a lot to say about you-know-what, it's not really a "sex manual." It's about strategies for living virtuously and profitably when it comes to matters of the heart (and other parts of the body). The Sanskrit word काम (*kāma*) means "desire," which is one of three purposes of human life according to Indian thinkers, along with material goods (अर्थ, *artha*) and virtue (धर्म, *dharma*).[1] The sentence we're looking at in this lesson is from the opening portion of the text, which explains why a treatise about desire is necessary. Our author, Vātsyāyana (not the Vātsyāyana from Lesson 3), argues that desire is a natural part of our lives and is intertwined with other purposes. But desire also requires effort and investigation to pursue well, so we can't just leave things to fate. And, for that reason, we should seriously study all kinds of relationships between human beings.

5.2.1 *Visarga* Sandhi: Changes before Vowels, Semi-Vowels, and Voiced Consonants

> **KEY POINTS:** If you see an "o" at the end of a noun, check whether it could have been a *visarga*. This will help you identify the case. Also, watch out for dropped *visargas* before the common quotation signal, इति (*iti*).

In our first lesson, we learned about the *visarga*, that little puff of air in योगः (*yogaḥ*), which sounds like *yoga*-hah. In Lesson 2, we learned that this sound changes when it comes into contact with three kinds of consonants, turning into an "s" sound, or a sibilant, as in श् (*ś*) before च (*ca*). Now, we will learn about when it transforms into an ओ (*o*). There are two ways this change can happen, both of which occur when the *visarga* follows the short अ (*a*), just as in योगः (*yogaḥ*). Suppose we add the verb we learned in Lesson 4 to the end of our sentence from Lesson 2, a verb you now understand is often optional:

1. Pandit point: Many also add a fourth, मोक्ष (*mokṣa*), or "liberation." This is an end to the ongoing cycle of life, suffering, death, and rebirth to which we're all bound.

योगश् चित्तवृत्तिनिरोधो ऽस्ति ।
yogaś cittavṛttinirodho 'sti.

In this example, the *visarga* in निरोधः (*nirodhaḥ*) is followed by the अ (*a*) in अस्ति (*asti*), which is then "chased away." That's when the "Sanskrit apostrophe" (ऽ) appears.[2]

Another transformation happens when the short अ (*a*) and *visarga* combination encounter certain consonants or semi-vowels. We've learned about semi-vowels already (you can look at the consonants table in Appendix 1 to jog your memory). Now, we'll learn about consonants known as *voiced* consonants. Voicing is the sound your vocal cords make when you utter a consonant. Try this: put your hand lightly on your throat and say "growl." You should feel a vibration. Then do the same while you say "kitten." You won't feel the same vibration. Table 22 updates our familiar table of consonants to identify which are voiced (+V) and which are unvoiced (-V).

Table 22. Consonants in transliteration, with voicing and aspiration

Point of Articulation	Consonants					Semi-Vowels	Sibilants	ह
Voice/ aspirated	-V / - A	-V / + A	+V / - A	+V / + A	+V / - A	+V / - A	- V / + A	+V / + A
Guttural	क ka	ख kha	ग ga	घ gha	ङ ṅa			ह ha
Palatal	च ca	छ cha	ज ja	झ jha	ञ ña	य ya	श śa	
Retroflex	ट ṭa	ठ ṭha	ड ḍa	ढ ḍha	ण ṇa	र ra	ष ṣa	
Dental	त ta	थ tha	द da	ध dha	न na	ल la	स sa	
Labial	प pa	फ pha	ब ba	भ bha	म ma	व va		

2. Pandit point: This is called an अवग्रह (*avagraha*). In this book, I follow the DHARMA transliteration guide and include a space before it, as in *nirodho 'sti* (Balogh and Griffiths 2020). Some Sanskritists prefer to elide the space: *nirodho'sti*.

Given this distinction, you can now understand a few more *visarga* patterns. Check out Table 23 and then the summary afterward.

Table 23. *Visarga* sandhi before vowels, semi-vowels, and voiced consonants

Visarga & Vowel	Initial Sound		*Visarga* Change?	Initial Sound Change?	Example
अः (*aḥ*)	voiced consonant (*g/gh*, etc.)	→	ओ (o)	none	rāmaḥ gacchati → rāmo gacchati रामः गच्छति → रामो गच्छति
अः (*aḥ*)	semi-vowel		ओ (o)	none	nirodhaḥ yogaḥ → nirodho yogaḥ निरोधः योगः → निरोधो योगः
अः (*aḥ*)	अ (*a*)		ओ (o)	changes to *avagraha*	dharmaḥ arthaḥ → dharmo 'rthaḥ धर्मः अर्थः → धर्मो ऽर्थः
अः (*aḥ*)	non-*a* vowels		अ (*a*)	none	dharmaḥ iti → dharma iti धर्मः इति → धर्म इति

In other words, much of the time, the ending अः (*-aḥ*) will change to ो (*-o*), and sometimes, an initial अ (*a*) disappears, replaced with ऽ. What happens in the other cases? You've already learned about the change to an "s" sound, or sibilant. When अः (*-aḥ*) meets any other vowel, like इ (*i*) or उ (*u*), the *visarga* drops, leaving अ (*-a*). Since the discourse particle इति (*iti*) often comes at the end of sentences, this is an important place to keep an eye out for sandhi.

5.2.2 The Genitive Case

> **KEY POINT:** The genitive often signals possession, and in English, the word "of" usually does the same thing.

In Lesson 3, I introduced you to the genitive. We saw that in English, we often use the preposition "of" to communicate its meaning, or else a possessive apostrophe, as in the underlined words in these examples:

1. The horse of Rāma travels. Rāma's horse travels.
2. The desire of the Buddha is *nirvāṇa*. The Buddha's desire is *nirvāṇa*.
3. There is cessation of actions. Actions's cessation occurs.

In Sanskrit, as we've emphasized, word order is fairly fluid because it's through how these words are formed that we know *what* belongs to *whom*. However, as we saw in Lesson 3, the genitive usually precedes the word that it modifies. Here's how the same sentences could be written in Sanskrit, with the genitive form underlined:[3]

1. रामस्य अश्वः गच्छति ।
*rāmasya aśvaḥ gacchati.

Rāma's horse travels.

2. बुद्धस्य प्रयोजनम् निर्वाणम् अस्ति ।
*buddhasya prayojanam nirvāṇam asti.

The Buddha's goal is *nirvāṇa*.

3. कर्मणाम् निरोधः भवति ।
*karmaṇām nirodhaḥ bhavati.

There is cessation of actions.

Below are tables showing the *declension* for the two nouns in our vocabulary list. Notice that the patterns of their endings, in bold, are not quite identical. Declension patterns vary in nouns because of two things: first,

3. By now, you know enough sandhi to transform each of the three sentences into the version you'd see in print. Try it and check your answers at the end of this lesson.

the grammatical gender (masculine, feminine, neuter), and second, the different endings in their stem (the most fundamental form). Here, both are neuter, but कर्मन् (*karman*) ends in -*an* and भद्र (*bhadra*) ends in -*a*. This means they follow different patterns. I use the preposition "of" to convey that these are genitive.

Table 24. *a*-stem neuter, genitive (भद्र/*bhadra*)

Singular	Dual	Plural
भद्रस्य bhadra**sya** (of prosperity)	भद्रयोः bhadra**yoḥ** (of two prosperities)	भद्राणाम् bhadr**āṇām** (of prosperities)

Actually, if you know the neuter भद्र (*bhadra*), you also know how to decline a-stem masculine nouns like योग (*yoga*). Just add the bolded endings, as in Table 25.

Table 25. *a*-stem masculine, genitive (योग/*yoga*)

Singular	Dual	Plural
योगस्य yoga**sya** (of yoga)	योगयोः yoga**yoḥ** (of two yogas)	योगानाम् yog**ānām** (of yogas)

The pattern for nouns ending in -*an* is a little different.

Table 26. *an*-stem neuter, genitive (कर्मन्/*karman*)

Singular	Dual	Plural
कर्मणः karmaṇ**aḥ** (of action)	कर्मणोः karmaṇ**oḥ** (of two actions)	कर्मणाम् karmaṇ**ām** (of actions)

These different patterns are similar to how words in English change based on number. To make "dog" plural, we add "-s" to form "dogs." But the plural of "elf" is *not* "elfs" but "elves"—we add "-es" *and* we change the spelling from "f" to "v"! However, many "deer" are just "deer." These different patterns become second nature after a lot of exposure, especially if you learn a language as a child. What makes Sanskrit easy to learn in some sense is that there are regularities based on the grammatical gender and a noun's form (whether an *-a* or *-an* stem). For now, notice the differences and see if you can identify the declension in the sample lesson.

5.2.3 Nasal Sandhi: न् (*n*) to ण् (*ṇ*)

> **KEY POINT:** The nasal sound changes based on what sounds precede it, which can make declined words look different when endings are applied.

You might have also noticed that the singular genitive for the word कर्मन् (*karman*) is कर्मणः (*karmaṇaḥ*), while the plural genitive of भद्र (*bhadra*) is भद्राणाम् (*bhadrāṇām*). Why not कर्मनः (*karmanaḥ*) or भद्रानाम् (*bhadrānām*)? This is because of a sandhi rule about dentals and retroflexes (go back to Lesson 1 if you need a refresher on the points of articulation): certain sounds "trigger" changes in later sounds. We can think about this as our tongues being lazy—or positively, as preserving energy. When we pronounce words, we'd like to do as little movement as possible while still distinguishing sounds. So, when certain retroflex sounds occur, unless our tongue has to move somewhere else when it gets to the "n" sound, it will choose the retroflex version rather than the dental. (This is like how our sibilants will change, as we saw in Lesson 2.) However, this only happens with certain sounds *after* the "n." For instance, if we are going to move our tongue to a dental like त् (*t*), we might as well make an effort with न् (*n*). And if another sound intervenes that requires our tongue to move, it blocks the change. As well, if न् (*n*) is the *final* sound in a word, like in कर्मन् (*karman*), then there's no change.

If this sounds like a lot to remember, a couple of points. First, we can make this clearer using a table (see Table 27). I have underlined the trigger sounds and, when relevant, put the *blocker sound* in italics. And second, as you see more vocabulary and pronounce more words, these patterns will become natural through exposure. So don't worry about committing these all to memory unless you want to. Focus on understanding how the sounds are produced.

Table 27. Dental and retroflex nasal sandhi

Trigger Sound	Intervening Sound	Sounds After न्	What Happens to न्?	Example
	vowels; *anusvāra*; gutturals; labials; ह् य् व्	vowels; न् म् य् व्	ण्	Rāmāyaṇa रामायण lakṣaṇa लक्षण
ऋ् (ṛ) र् (r) ष् (ṣ)	vowels; *anusvāra*; gutturals; labials; ह् य् व्	consonants; semi-vowels other than न् म् य् व्	न्	kūrvanti कूर्वन्ति
	palatal; cerebral; dental	not relevant- *blocker* present	न्	darśana दर्शन

5.2.4 Intransitive Verbs: Reminder

> **KEY POINT:** When you read a Sanskrit sentence, focus on the verb first. Then, see if there is a subject (in the nominative) that matches its number. There may or may not be an object, depending on the verb.

One last thing: in our example sentences, we've followed this pattern: subject, object, verb. But not all verbs must have an explicit object of action, as we saw in Lesson 3. That's the case for verbs like "to exist" and "to occur" in English and the 2P √अस् (*as*) and 1P √भू (*bhū*) in Sanskrit, which are intransitive. A transitive verb *trans*fers the action to the object, as when Leonardo takes the ball. The ball receives the action of taking.

But saying, “Leonardo takes,” leaves us hanging—what does he take? In the case of an *in*transitive verb, we have no such expectation for an object. For example, describing a pot, I might say:

Example
घटो ऽस्ति ।

ghaṭo 'sti.

The pot is. (= The pot exists.)

While I can add an adjective (more on these in Lesson 9—for now, notice they match in gender, number, and case), that adjective isn't receiving the action in the way that the ball does when Leonardo takes it. It's a predicate, giving information about the subject, as we saw in Lesson 4.

Example
घटो नीलो ऽस्ति ।

ghaṭo nīlo 'sti.

The pot is blue.

5.2.5 Exocentric Compounds

> **KEY POINT:** Always check whether a compound describes something possessed by another subject, whether explicit or implicit, in the sentence.

When we learned about the *determinative compound* in Lesson 2, I introduced it using English terminology, although I mentioned in a footnote that Sanskrit grammatical terms can be very helpful since they often illustrate the concept they describe. The *exocentric compound* is a good example of this. In Sanskrit, it's called a *bahuvrīhi* (बहुव्रीहि), which is a compound of two words: “many” (बहु, *bahu*) and “rice” (व्रीहि, *vrīhi*). But the compound doesn't refer to a big pile of rice—instead, it's a term for someone who has a lot of rice. In ancient India, this would have been a wealthy person. An English equivalent to बहुव्रीहि (*bahuvrīhi*) is "moneybags," a person who has a lot of money—which they used to store in bags, back when money wasn't almost entirely electronic. We often use these kinds of compounds in English, even without knowing it: redheads and baldheads aren't heads rolling around with or without hair, but they are people who *have* red heads or bald heads. In all of these cases, something else *possesses* what the compound refers to. Sometimes, that other thing is stated explicitly in the sentence, but often, especially in Sanskrit, it isn't. So, we need to figure out whether we're talking about a pile of rice or a *person who owns* a pile of rice.

One way to determine whether our compound is an exocentric compound is to look at the verb in the sentence. Or, if it's a nominal sentence without an explicit verb, we look at what the compound is describing. For instance, in English, consider these sentences:

1. The red coat is fraying.
2. The redcoat has charged up the hill.

In the first sentence, "red coat" refers to an actual piece of clothing since we're describing the material. In the second sentence, since clothing can't move on its own, we interpret the word "redcoat" as *the soldier wearing a redcoat*—this is what has charged up the hill.

There's another way to identify whether a compound is an exocentric compound, which requires paying attention to the grammatical gender of the last word (the "head") in the compound. Since exocentric compounds modify other things, their grammatical gender will match whatever thing they modify. In other words, in Sanskrit, if the "redcoat" refers to a female British soldier, it will have a feminine ending. And that's so even if the word "coat" has a neuter or masculine ending in the dictionary. Or, more abstractly, if the ending of the last word in the compound is different than the word's gender in the dictionary, you have an exocentric compound.

5.2.6 Indeclinables: Negation

KEY POINT: Words that do not decline or conjugate, like the negation न (*na*) before a verb, and the "Sanskrit quotation mark" इति (*iti*), are indeclinables.

In Lesson 3, you learned how verbs work in the present tense. But we didn't talk about how to negate a verb or say that the main action is *not* occurring. In English, we often use two words, "do not" or "does not," as in:

1. The horse of Rāma travels. The horse of Rāma *does not* travel.

3. The cessation of actions occurs. The cessation of actions *does not* occur.

Sanskrit is economical, in contrast. A single word, न (*na*), communicates that the action isn't happening. And, unlike English, there's no need to change anything about the verb (like dropping the "s" from "travels" to "does not travel"). Simply place न (*na*) before the verb (try it in the example sentences above). Watch for one thing: the negation doesn't have to be right in front of the verb. It can be separated by the subject and object (or predicate) of the sentence:

Pattern

negation subject predicate **verb**

Example

न योगश् चित्तवृत्तिनिरोधो **ऽस्ति** ।

na yogaś cittavṛttinirodho **'sti**

Yoga **is not** the cessation of the mind's activity.

Because the negation does not change according to number and other factors, like nouns do, it's called an *indeclinable*.

Another indeclinable in our reading is used to mark quotes: इति (*iti*). Sanskrit today is printed in books, often including commas, periods, and other punctuation marks. But originally, it was written on long palm leaves without much punctuation. There were no commas and only sometimes a *daṇḍa* (literally meaning "stick")—the punctuation mark । used to signal a full stop, typically found where modern editions would use periods. And there were certainly no quotation marks to identify when someone was speaking. Instead, Sanskrit uses the word इति (*iti*) to show the end of a person's speech or thought. That requires us to figure out where the beginning of the quoted material is in the sentence. (Usually, it's a complete thought and clear from context.) One way इति (*iti*) works is to attribute a thought or statement to someone.

Pattern

subject object (or predicate) verb *iti* name

Example

योगश् चित्तवृत्तिनिरोध **इति** पतञ्जलिः ।

yogaś cittavṛttinirodha[4] **iti** patañjaliḥ.

Yoga is cessation of the mind's activity, according to Patañjali.

"Yoga is cessation of the mind's activity"—Patañjali.

We can either read इति (*iti*) as "according to" or use punctuation like quotation marks and a dash to show that we're working with a quote. The main thing is to understand that this indeclinable word is telling us how to interpret the words before it.[5]

---

4. Pandit point: That slippery *visarga* has disappeared here because of sandhi when it confronts a vowel.

5. Pandit point: This makes it a *discourse marker*, or a word that isn't referring to things in the world but to the language itself. Discourse markers are (usually) small words that pack a lot of information about what's going on in a sentence. They're worth paying attention to.

5.2.7 Prefixes

> **KEY POINT:** If you can't find a word in a Sanskrit dictionary, check whether it has a prefix. If so, look up the main word without the prefix.

One last little bit to know. A very little bit, in fact, since *prefixes* are small parts of words. They attach to the beginning of words to modify their meaning. This happens in English, too:

1. *Noun prefixes*: The pizza was ordinary. The pizza was *extra*ordinary.
2. *Verb prefixes*: The queen built a castle. The queen *re*built a castle.

If we know the meaning of "extra-" and "re-", then we can usually predict what the meaning of a word will be when these prefixes are attached to them.[6] The same is true for Sanskrit. Our vocabulary list has the prefix निष् (*niṣ*-), which means "without" or "lacking" when it's in front of a noun or a verb. A second meaning is "away from" or "out," which we see in a well-known word: निर्वाण (*nirvāṇa*), meaning "blowing out" from a form of the verb √वा (*vā*) and the prefix निर् (*nir*-).[7] Understanding prefixes helps us predict what words mean when these terms are combined. Another reason to know about prefixes in Sanskrit is that dictionary entries typically put the prefixed versions of the words as subentries. This would be like an English dictionary putting "extraordinary" under the entry "ordinary." Once you recognize that "extra-" is a prefix, to look

6. Pandit point: I say *usually* because there are always exceptions. For instance, "flammable" means something easily lit on fire. But so does the word "*in*flammable," even though, based on how "visible" and "*in*visible" work, we might think they are opposites.

7. Pandit point: This prefix is spelled differently depending on the word it is prefixed with, as you might expect, given what you know about sandhi. So you will also see निश् (*niś*-), निस् (*nis*-), निर् (*nir*-), and निः (*niḥ*-). You might guess—and you'd be right—that these patterns have something to do with *visarga* sandhi.

up “extraordinary,” you’d turn the pages to (or type into your search bar) the word “ordinary.”

5.3 Putting Everything Together

न निष्कर्मणो भद्रम् अस्तीति वात्स्यायनः।

na niṣkarmaṇo bhadram astīti vātsyāyanaḥ.

The first word of our reading is the indeclinable negation, telling you that there is a main verb that is negated. Your knowledge of vowel sandhi from the past lessons will help you identify the main verb and recognize what tiny word it has become connected to. You also know enough about compounds to be able to interpret the genitive form of one of our vocabulary words as belonging to a person.

A parallel English sentence might help you transition from the grammar of the Sanskrit sentence to a more understandable English. Take the sentence:

Example

Fear that belongs to a redcoat does not exist.

In English, this is awkward. It’d be simpler to say:

A redcoat has no fear.

Both sentences express roughly the same idea about the relationship between redcoats and fear. But the first sentence takes “fear” as the subject of a verb (“exist”), whereas the second makes “redcoat” the subject of a verb (“have”). In our reading, we also have something that does not exist:

Example

न निष्कर्मणो भद्रम् असतीति वात्स्यायनः।

na niṣkarmaṇo bhadram astīti vātsyāyanaḥ.

bhadra belonging to *niṣkarman* does not exist *iti vātsyāyanaḥ*

And while *niṣkarman* means "lacking activity," consider whether *bhadra* is something that we'd say a lack of activity has on its own or whether someone or something lacks activity, like "redcoat," an adjective for something unstated in the sentence.

5.4 About the Reading: Romance Is Hard Work

The statement attributed to Vātsyāyana emphasizes the importance of hard work. He's responding to an imagined conversation partner who argues that since everything depends on chance—or fate—there's no point trying to live any particular way. After all, what happens, happens! But Vātsyāyana thinks this is a poor excuse, and, in our reading and the rest of his introduction, argues that people need to work hard to get what they want and regulate their desires. It's with this background in mind that we should read the rest of the text, famous for sex positions and romantic advice. The *Kāmasūtra* isn't a handbook for unbridled hedonism, but it recognizes that self-control is important even in seeking out sensual satisfaction.[8] This means choosing suitable partners, implementing strategies that might take time to come to fruition, and being aware of social norms—and how to manipulate them to one's best interest.

The *Kāmasūtra*, then, is not unlike the *Yogasūtra* in its emphasis on discipline. And both are about much more than "positions," whether yogic or sensual. Educated people of ancient India would have read both texts, as well as the *Upaniṣad* we were introduced to in the last lesson. For more on the *Kāmasūtra*, see McConnachie (2008) and Doniger (2016).

8. See Doniger (2016, 57–61).

Self-Quiz Answers

1. रामस्य अश्वः गच्छति → रामस्याश्वो गच्छति
rāmasya aśvaḥ gacchati → rāmasyāśvo gacchati

2. बुद्धस्य कामम् निर्वाणम् अस्ति → बुद्धस्य कामं निर्वाणम् अस्ति
buddhasya kāmam nirvāṇam asti → buddhasya kāmaṃ nirvāṇam asti

3. कर्मणाम् निरोधः भवति → कर्मणाम् निरोधो भवति
karmaṇām nirodhaḥ bhavati → karmaṇām nirodho bhavati

Lesson 6

Reading: Chāndogya Upaniṣad 6.8.7

तत् त्वम् असि श्वेतकेतो ।

tat tvam asi śvetaketo.

Points of Interest For

The Curious: How demonstrative pronouns work is the central idea you need to understand in this lesson (6.2.2), as you have the verb from Lesson 4 and can check out the table to understand the second-person pronoun.

The Yoga Aficionado: The end of 6.2.3 is important for reading printed Devanāgarī; don't skip it.

The Scholar: See the online translation solutions for discussion of some controversy over the little word तत् (*tat*).

6.1 Vocabulary

Devanāgarī	Transliteration	Part of Speech	Translation
इदम्	idam	pn.	this
एतद्	etad	pn.	this
तद्	tad	pn.	that
अस्मद्	asmad	1 pn.	I
युष्मद्	yuṣmad	2 pn.	you
श्वेतकेतु	śvetaketu	masc. proper name	Śvetaketu
हे	he	ptc.	Hey!; oh! (direct address)

6.2 Grammar Notes

KEY POINTS: Pronouns in Sanskrit carry a lot of information by their gender, number, and case. Second-personal pronouns like "you" and demonstrative pronouns like "it" both decline as we've learned nouns do.

Hey, reader! If you've been looking for an exciting lesson, this is it!

In those sentences, I've employed all the grammatical concepts we'll cover in this lesson. First, I addressed you directly with "Hey, reader." In Sanskrit, that kind of statement—direct address—would be in the vocative case. Then, in a sentence using the second-personal pronoun, "you," I used two different pronouns to refer to the lesson. Unless you're a stickler for grammar, you probably weren't focused on the pronouns I used ("it," "this") and how they are able to refer to the lesson. Called *demonstrative pronouns*, they let us talk about objects at various distances from the speaker—*this* thing here, *that* thing way over there.

At the end of this lesson, you'll have the tools to read part of another "Great Sentence" (महावाक्य, *mahāvākya*) like we read in Lesson 4. This sentence appears in the *Chāndogya Upaniṣad* and, like our other *mahāvākya*, deals with who we are in relationship to reality, a big topic condensed into three little words: तत् त्वम् असि (*tat tvam asi*).[1]

6.2.1 Personal Pronouns: Second Person

> **KEY POINT:** The Sanskrit second-person pronoun is equivalent to the English "you," except that it allows us to say "you two" and "you many" in a single-word form.

English speakers have a distinct disadvantage when it comes to the second-person pronoun, or "you." Many English dialects lack a grammatical marker to distinguish "you," *singular*, from "you," *plural*. To make up for this, regional variations arise in the United States: *yinz* in Pittsburgh, *youse guys* in Philadelphia or New Jersey. In the Southern regions, *y'all* have one of the most widely adapted forms of the second-person pronoun plural.

Sanskrit has many forms of the second-person pronoun, including a plural. As we've already seen, pronouns are case declined. In Lesson 4, we learned about the first-person pronoun, whose stem form is अस्मद् (*asmad*) but declines in the nominative singular as अहम् (*aham*). The second-person pronoun is like the first-person pronoun. Its stem form is similar, युष्मद् (yuṣmad), and the endings in its paradigm are also similar. Below are both nominative paradigms so you can see their

1. Pandit point: Strictly speaking, this sentence and the other sentence from the *Upaniṣads* is from a kind of Sanskrit known as "Vedic." This earlier kind of Sanskrit has some grammatical features that Classical Sanskrit loses, like accents. For our purposes, I use these two very short sentences to illustrate some common features, but there's some controversy over the meaning of this sentence, which depends on the particularities of Vedic grammar. See Brereton (1986). The University of Texas at Austin Linguistics Department has a nice introduction to Vedic Sanskrit online. See the online resources in the Introduction to this volume.

similarities. The full paradigms for these and all the declensions in this lesson are in Appendix 1. If you remember from Lesson 4, the ते (*te*) in नमस्ते (*namaste*) is a shortened form called an *enclitic*, which is listed in Appendix 1, too. It's the dative form of the second-person pronoun.

Table 28. Second-person pronoun, nominative (युष्मद्/*yuṣmad*)

	Singular	Dual	Plural
Nominative (subject)	त्वम् (tv**am**) - you	युवाम् (yuv**ām**) - you two	यूयम् (yūy**am**) - you all

Table 29. First-person pronoun, nominative (अस्मद्/asmad)

	Singular	Dual	Plural
Nominative (subject)	अहम् (ah**am**) - I	आवाम् (āv**ām**) - we two	वयम् (vay**am**) - we

Neither pronoun is gendered, so you only need to learn to recognize these three paradigms, unlike the pronouns we'll learn next, which all decline in masculine, feminine, and neuter. Also, none of these pronouns have a vocative form. They aren't used for direct address.

6.2.2 Demonstrative Pronouns

KEY POINT: Pay attention to the grammatical information conveyed by demonstrative pronouns to identify their referent.

Pronouns let us refer to things quickly and concisely, whether we're pointing out something that we see ("Hey, look at *that*!") or we're pointing out something already said ("*That* is what Shakespeare said in Sonnet 18.")[2]

2. Pandit point: The Sanskrit word for a pronoun is सर्वनाम (*sarvanāma*), a compound that means "name for everything." That's because a pronoun can be used to "name," or refer to, anything you want.

In contrast to personal pronouns, which are used to stand in for the person speaking ("*I* am walking here!") or a person who is the object of an action ("I'm talking to *you*"), demonstrative pronouns stand in for a third thing, some object. Whether "that" refers to a brightly colored bird in the trees, a stanza of a sonnet, or something else depends on context. In English, pronoun forms change depending on number: from "this" to "these." In Sanskrit, pronoun forms also reflect number, but, as you will expect by now, they also vary depending on grammatical gender and case.

Like nouns, pronouns have three numbers—singular, dual, and plural—and three genders—masculine, neuter, and feminine. And, too, they have eight cases, including the nominative, accusative, and genitive, which we've already seen. When a pronoun appears in Sanskrit, we have more clues about its referent than we would in English. Suppose you and I are hiking, and I say:

> Look at <u>that</u>!

You know I want to draw your attention to something. It's probably one thing since I didn't say "those." But is it a bird, a turtle, an amazing vista? In contrast, if I were to say the same thing in Sanskrit, it could amount to:

> Look at <u>that-single-feminine-object</u>!

Or instead:

> Look at <u>that-single-neuter-object</u>!

Since nouns have grammatical genders, you have more information about what I'm pointing to: the name for it will match in grammatical gender. Sanskrit also has another clue. Depending on how far away the object is—either physically or, in the case of discourse, how long ago the thing was said—we use different pronouns.

Figure 3 illustrates the relationship between these three common pronouns as concentric circles. The pronoun एतद् (*etad*) is used for nearby objects, इदम् (*idam*) for things a bit farther away, and तद् (*tad*) for things even farther away from the speaker.[3]

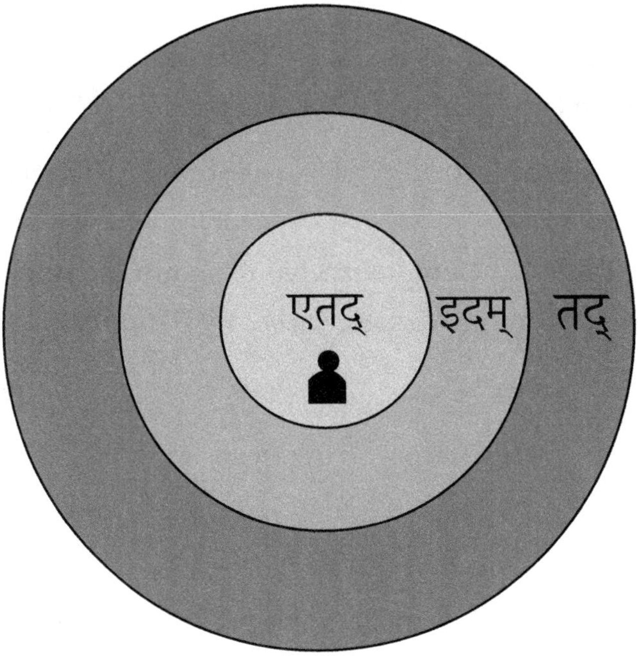

Figure 3. एतद् (*etad*), इदम् (*idam*), तद् (*tad*)

Though each of the three pronouns has three paradigms, one for each grammatical gender, let's not try to learn all nine at once. Instead, let's just focus on the nominative and accusative cases. That's because we have a two-for-one deal going with these for the neuter. Below are the three pronouns in their neuter nominative *and* accusative cases. Neuter nouns are typically the same form in nominative and accusative.

3. Pandit point: You will sometimes see the stem form of two of these pronouns spelled as एतत् (*etat*) and तत् (*tat*) and given in grammars in root form as एत- (*eta*-) and त- (*ta*-). That's for reasons concerning how stems, which don't occur in ordinary language, are reconstructed for grammars.

Table 30. Demonstrative pronoun, neuter, nominative/accusative (तद्/*tad*)

	Singular	Dual	Plural
Nominative	तत् t**at** (that)	ते t**e** (those two)	तानि t**āni** (those)
Accusative	तत् t**at** (that)	ते t**e** (those two)	तानि t**āni** (those)

Table 31. Demonstrative pronoun, neuter, nominative/accusative (इदम्/*idam*)

	Singular	Dual	Plural
Nominative	इदम् id**am** (that)	इमे im**e** (those two)	इमानि im**āni** (those)
Accusative	इदम् id**am** (that)	इमे im**e** (those two)	इमानि im**āni** (those)

Table 32. Demonstrative pronoun, neuter, nominative/accusative (एतद् /*etad*)

	Singular	Dual	Plural
Nominative	एतत् et**at** (this)	एते et**e** (these two)	एतानि et**āni** (these)
Accusative	एतत् et**at** (this)	एते et**e** (these two)	एतानि et**āni** (these)

Finally, let's look at the masculine form of the demonstrative pronoun तद् (*tad*), whose nominative singular form सः (*saḥ*) is very common.

Table 33. Demonstrative pronoun, masculine, nominative/accusative (तद्/*tad*)

	Singular	Dual	Plural
Nominative	सः saḥ (he)	तौ t**au** (he two)	ते t**e** (those, they)
Accusative	तम् t**am** (him)	तौ t**au** (him two)	तान् t**ān** (those, them)

You might notice that the form is very similar to the *a*-stem masculine declension we learned earlier in Lesson 3 for योग (*yoga*). And the *visarga* rule that applies before vowels applies here, too, which is why the form in some sentences may be स (*sa*), not सः (*saḥ*).[4]

6.2.3 Vowel Sandhi: Dissimilar Vowels

> **KEY POINT:** The principle of vowel strengthening is that we "add" अ (*a*) to vowels in a regular pattern. This happens between words and within words.

In this book so far, I've given you examples of sandhi in Sanskrit, but we haven't talked much about the underlying reasons for the sound changes. That's intentional—there's quite a lot we could cover, and there are other resources available. Still, this is a good point at which to introduce you to an important concept in Sanskrit phonology: *vowel strength*. In Lesson 1, you learned about short and long vowel pairs. Some of these vowels are *simple*—basic sounds that involve nothing other than opening your mouth in a particular way and expelling sound. It's like when the doctor asks you to open your mouth and say "Ah" as she puts in a tongue depressor. There's no moving your tongue against your teeth, etc. These vowels are below.

Table 34. Simple vowels

Short Vowel	Long Vowel
अ a - b**u**t	आ ā - b**aw**dy
इ i - b**i**t	ई ī - b**ee**
उ u - p**u**t	ऊ ū - p**oo**l

4. Pandit point: This pronoun behaves unusually before consonants, however. In the masculine singular, the *visarga* drops before consonants, too.

Now, with simple vowels, we can understand the relationship between vowel sounds in another way: in terms of how strong or weak they are. Vowel strength isn't measured in pounds or kilograms but in अ's. We can take any of these simple vowels and add an अ (*a*) to the beginning to strengthen it. We can do this twice, in fact (but no more). It's a bit like math with sounds. Take the simple vowel, इ (*i*). We can strengthen it twice:

Example

Strong: अ (*a*) + इ (*i*) → ए (*e*)

Strongest: अ (*a*) + ए (*e*) → ऐ (*ai*)

This means that for each simple vowel, we have three levels—called *grades*—of strength: normal, strong, and strongest or इ (*i*), ए (*e*), ऐ (*ai*), in this example.[5] Notice that "adding" अ (*a*) to itself takes *two additions* before it strengthens. And we can't get any stronger than आ (*ā*).

Table 35. Vowel grades according to strength

Normal Simple Vowel	Strong अ (a) + Normal	Strongest अ (a) + Medium
अ (*a*)	अ (*a*)	आ (*ā*)
आ (*ā*)	आ (*ā*)	आ (*ā*)
इ (*i*) / ई (*ī*)	ए (*e*)	ऐ (*ai*)
उ (*u*) / ऊ (*ū*)	ओ (*o*)	औ (*au*)
ऋ (*ṛ*)	अर् (*ar*)	आर् (*ār*)[6]

5. Pandit point: The two stronger levels have Sanskrit terms that are very common in textbooks: गुण (*guṇa*), meaning "secondary degree," and वृद्धि (*vṛddhi*), meaning "increase."

6. Pandit point: For simplicity, we're skipping the ॠ (*ṝ*) and ऌ (*ḷ*) in this book. The first has the same strengthening as *ṛ*, while the second would be अल् (*al*).

Why does this matter? Well, some of the regular sound changes in Sanskrit occur through this kind of addition. This happens between words and within words.

For example, the words छान्दोग्य (*chāndogya*) and उपणिषत् (*upaniṣat*),[7] when put into compound, combine अ (*a*) + उ (*u*), which results in ओ (*o*). In compound, it's spelled छान्दोग्योपणिषत् (*chāndogyo**o**paniṣat*). And sometimes vowels strengthen on their own, as when declension or conjugation patterns involve strengthening. So, it's useful to understand this idea. It helps you identify what they look like in their weakened forms by "subtracting." For example, the 8P verb √कृ (*kṛ*), "to do," or "to make," is करोति (*karoti*) in the present indicative third person singular—we'll see that verb again in Lesson 7. Based on your understanding of the verb ending and strengthening patterns, you can work out some of how this happens. Try it! Hint: remove the ending -ओति (*-oti*) and focus on the root to stem change.

One more vowel change is important to know, which is when a few vowels change into semi-vowels (य, र, व). Only five vowels do this, and these are easily remembered as pairs: इ/ई (*i/ī*), उ/ऊ (*u/ū*), ऋ (*ṛ*).[8] Each of these will turn into its corresponding semi-vowel (य, व, र) when it encounters another vowel (or diphthong). The following vowels will stay the same while the previous vowel changes to a semi-vowel.

---

7. Pandit point: The final त् (*t*) is because this is the form for the nominative case, not the stem.

8. Pandit point: Remember that ऋ (*ṛ*) has a stronger partner, but we aren't worrying about it much in this book.

Table 36. Vowel sandhi to corresponding semi-vowel

Vowel		Corresponding Semi-Vowel	Example
इ/ई (*i/ī*)	→	य् (*y*)	iti arthaḥ → ity arthaḥ इति अर्थः → इत्यर्थः
उ/ऊ (*u/ū*)		व् (*v*)	śvetaketu idam → śvetaketv idam श्वेतकेतु इदम् → श्वेतकेत्विदम्
ऋ (*ṛ*)		र् (*r*)	kartṛ etat = kartr etat कर्तृ एतत् = कर्त्रेतत्

Finally, you're probably noticing something else strange going on. Instead of keeping the words separate in the Devanāgarī, they are combining: इत्यर्थः (but we transliterate it as *ity arthaḥ*). This is perfectly normal and another reason why learning to read Sanskrit in Devanāgarī can take some time. Until this lesson, we have been separating words to make it easier for you, which means you've gotten used to seeing the stop mark (*virāma*) at the end of words, like इत्य् अर्थः or योगश् चित्ति. However, most printed texts do not do this. Typically, they join words together even when there are consonants between them: इत्यर्थः or योगश्चित्ति. In contrast, words ending in the *anusvāra* (e.g., मित्रं) or the *visarga* (e.g., योगः) are left separate.

When you read Devanāgarī, then, it's important to consider why two words are joined: Is it because they are in compound, because of sandhi, or because of printing conventions? However, when *transliterating* Sanskrit texts, typically we insert spaces between word boundaries where there is consonant sandhi. (The convention is not to remove sandhi, however, so the sandhi remains in place: *ity arthaḥ*, not *iti arthaḥ*.) We'll start printing Devanāgarī script words together in the next lesson more often.

6.2.4 Vocative Case

KEY POINT: Vocatives let the speaker address someone (or something) directly.

Hey, reader! Don't give up yet, *reader*! This is the last section. The words in italics play a special role, direct address, which is our last topic. *Direct address* is when you're talking *to* rather than *about* someone. It's the difference between

1. The student reads the book.
2. Student! Read the book.[9]

Case-declined languages like Sanskrit employ the vocative case for nouns used for direct address.[10] Any noun can be declined in the vocative, though we most often see relational nouns (father, mother, daughter, son) and proper names (Sītā, Rāma) declined this way. How can you recognize a vocative? There are a few ways.

First, know that the vocative may be *precisely the same form* as the nominative, except that in the singular, it may drop the ending or strengthen the vowel in the stem form. The vocative is frequently used for a single person, so it could be the vocative when a proper name lacks an ending. (Of course, you need to check that other kinds of sandhi aren't present.) For instance, here are two ways to decline the name of Śvetaketu, the person in our reading:

1. श्वेतकेतुः (*śvetaketuḥ*) - masculine nominative singular
2. श्वेतकेतो (*śvetaketo*) - masculine vocative singular

---

9. Pandit point: In Sanskrit, there's another important difference. In sentence (1), the verb "reads" is in the present indicative, which we learned about in Lesson 3. In sentence (2), the verb is in the imperative mood, which we'll talk about in Lesson 13. In Sanskrit, these verbs have different conjugations, so they would be formed differently.

10. Pandit point: Sanskrit grammarians like Pāṇini don't consider this a proper case or विभक्ति (*vibhakti*). But we'll talk about it that way in this book. If you're curious about how the vocative works in Sanskrit and how grammarians have understood it, look at Chakrabarti (2016).

We haven't learned how to decline masculine nouns ending in *-u* just yet, but notice that the उ (*u*) ending in the stem form has been strengthened by the same rules we just learned. Now, following this same pattern, what do you think the vocative *might* be for a stem form that ends in इ (*i*)?

If a word in the vocative can be spelled exactly the same as a word in the nominative, the subject of a sentence, how can you recognize it? Look at the meaning of the sentence. When a word is used for direct address, it will not make sense as the subject or object of any verb. In a way, it's just hanging out, not connected to anything.[11] That's why they're separated from the rest of the sentence in English by commas or exclamation marks. In Sanskrit, they often appear at the beginning or end of sentences.

Finally, you will often see a Sanskrit particle before direct address: the particle हे (*he*). If you are an English speaker, this is easy to remember: it's like saying, "*He*y Rāma!" (Unlike "hey," हे (*he*) can be more formal, depending on the context.)

6.3 Putting Everything Together

तत् त्वम् असि श्वेतकेतो ।

tat tvam asi śvetaketo.

To read this lesson's sentence, you may want to review the conjugation of the 2P verb √अस् (*as*) from Lesson 4. Remember that a sentence using this verb, which means "to be," is expressing that one thing Y is another

11. Pandit point: Syntacticians, pragmaticians, and other linguists have lots to say on precisely what vocatives are and how they connect to sentences. Some argue they're like little sentences on their own. Bhartṛhari, a Sanskrit grammarian, is explicit that the vocative isn't part of the sentence meaning even when we're commanding someone, but his commentator Helarāja disagrees. See Chakrabarti (2016, 199).

thing X—in grammatical terms, the sentence is *predicating* X of Y. And in Sanskrit, the word order is usually:

Pattern

subject predicate verb

X Y is = X is Y

If I want to use pronouns to talk about what something is, I might say:

Example

एतानि सूत्राणि सन्ति ।

etāni sūtrāṇi santi.

These (*etāni*) are (*santi*) *sūtras* (*sūtrāṇi*).

I can even use two pronouns to talk about something:

Example

एतानि तानि सन्ति ।

etāni tāni santi.

These (*etāni*) are (*santi*) those (*tāni*).

Now, see if you can read this lesson's small Great Sentence!

6.4 About the Reading: Who Are You?

In Book Six of the *Chāndogya Upaniṣad*, a brahmin named Uddālaka Āruṇi is talking to his son, Śvetaketu. As a twelve-year-old boy, Śvetaketu had gone off to study the Vedas. Now he has returned twelve years later, pretty full of himself. So, his father asks him questions that show the young man he doesn't know quite as much as he thinks. Eventually, Śvetaketu realizes he needs help and asks his father to explain things to him. Uddālaka describes the origins of reality and the nature of the world as it exists today, continuing throughout several chapters.

By Chapter Eight of Book Six, the brahmin isn't only explaining the nature of the world around Śvetaketu but how this world is related to Śvetaketu himself. That means the sentence's pronoun तत् (*tat*) refers to something in their conversation. It's a pronoun that looks backward to the rest of the sentences—an *anaphoric* pronoun. One famous Sanskrit commentator, whom we've talked about before, Śaṅkara, argues that this sentence is identifying Śvetaketu with the world, which is Brahman, just like in the sentence in Lesson 4. Others, like the philosopher Madhva, disagree, saying it refers to something else. Who is right? We can't answer unless we read the rest of the sentences, and there are philosophical disputes over how to interpret these, too.

Let me tell you one of the more creative approaches, which shows the importance of sandhi in reading Sanskrit. In palm-leaf manuscripts, sentences in Sanskrit were strung together with little punctuation. A stop or *daṇḍa* (।) might appear only at the end of a section. So, without sandhi, this sentence and the sentence just before it reads:

स आत्मातत्त्वमसि (*sa ātmātattvamasi*)

As we have learned, the vowel आ (ā) can be the result of several vowel sandhi combinations:

अ + अ (*a* + *a*)
आ + अ (*ā* + *a*)
अ + आ (*a* + *ā*)
आ + आ (*ā* + *ā*)

Madhva thought it made the most sense to split these words apart this way:

स आत्मा । अतत् त्वम् असि । (*sa ātmā. atat tvam asi.*)

The first two words say, "This (masculine nominative singular) is the self" (see Lesson 10).[12] And by splitting sandhi, "that" (*tat*) becomes "non-that" (*a-tat*), since (*a*) is a prefix that means "not" or "non." Another philosopher, Viṣṇudāsa, gave twenty readings of just the three words तत् त्वम् असि (*tat tvam asi*)! But we'll leave things here for now.

Self-Quiz Answers

Answer to question about करोति: कृ → कर् by strengthening once. As for the rest, the verb ending for the third-person singular also involves strengthening. The stem कर् adds उ, which then takes strengthening to ओ, and the ending -ति is affixed.

Answer to question about vocative ending in इ (*i*): for masculine and feminine forms that end in इ (*i*) and उ (*u*), the forms are ए (*e*) and ओ (*o*). Neuter forms ending in these vowels work differently, and there are many other stem endings.

12. Pandit point: The word आत्मा (*ātmā*) is the masculine nominative singular form of आत्मन् (*ātman*), which makes the first sentence a nominal sentence. स (*sa*) is the same form but of the masculine demonstrative pronoun तद् (*tad*). It declines like योग (*yoga*), so you might suspect some *visarga* sandhi has happened here—and you'd be right.

Lesson 7

Reading: Arthaśāstra 7.9.12

यावदुपकरोति तावन्मित्रं
भवति ।
उपकारलक्षणं मित्रम् ।

yāvad upakaroti tāvan mitraṃ bhavati.
upakāralakṣaṇaṃ mitram.

Points of Interest For

The Curious: Focus on the relative-correlative construction to help you understand the structure of this reading.

The Yoga Aficionado: You may be familiar with the "four aims" (*puruṣārthas*); this reading is about one of them, *artha* or material prosperity; check out the information about the reading at the end to see how.

The Scholar: You might want to look ahead to 8.2.1 and then come back to the relative-correlative construction again since these are part of the same idea.

7.1 Vocabulary

Devanāgarī	Transliteration	Part of Speech	Translation
अर्थशास्त्र	arthaśāstra	masc. n., cpd.	*Treatise on Success* (title)
उपकार	upakāra	masc. n.	assistance, help
√कृ (+ उप)	√kṛ (+ upa)	v. (8P)	assist, help
तावत्	tāvat	correlative pn.	to the extent that
नीति	nīti	fem. n.	leadership; good conduct
पूर्वपक्ष	pūrvapakṣa	masc. n., cpd.	earlier position (in a debate, the opponent's view)
√बुध्	√budh	v. (1P)	understand, learn
√भू	√bhū	v. (1P)	to be, to exist
मित्र	mitra	neut. n.	friend, ally
यावत्	yāvat	rel. pn.	to the extent that
लक्षण	lakṣaṇa	neut. n.	characteristic, definition
विन्दसि	vindasi	2 sg., pres. indc. v. from √*vid* (6P)	you think (second person present indicative)

7.2 Grammar Notes

KEY POINT: Learning new verb conjugations, like the 8P in this lesson, is easier once you have confidence with the 1P conjugation introduced in Lesson 3.

Not all Sanskrit literature is abstract metaphysical speculation like we saw in the last lesson. Much of it is aimed at practical advice for living well, whether you are a king, a queen, or an ordinary Jane or Joe (or Draupadī or Devadatta). In this lesson and the next, we'll look at some thoughts about friendship. First, we'll read a definition of friendship written by Kauṭilya in the *Arthaśāstra*, or the *Treatise on Success*, as one translator renders the title. Its first word, *artha*, has a range of meanings, including "aim," "wealth," and "purpose," all of which are relevant to this political text.[1] Friendship in this context could include warm fuzzy feelings but was defined more pragmatically. Our lesson introduces some new verbs and the concept of *relative-correlative pairs*.

7.2.1 Introduction to Relative-Correlative Pairs

> **KEY POINT:** Pronouns in Sanskrit are frequently linked together. The *yāvat-tāvat* pairing is just one example.

Children of the 1980s grew up with a public service announcement on U.S. TV which said, with a little jingle, "The more you know . . ." It's not a complete sentence—hearing it, we wondered, the more you know, what? This is a *dependent* or *relative clause*, not an independent sentence, and it requires another clause to make it grammatical, like:

Example

1. The more you know, the more you understand.

This kind of construction happens a lot in pithy sayings:

Example

2. The bigger they are, the harder they fall.

---

1. Pandit point: While I say "written by" Kauṭilya, more strictly speaking, he is the compiler and arranger of the text. For a translation of the text and copious scholarly notes, see Olivelle (2016).

These constructions pair two clauses together, linking the information in the first clause—about some thing—to the information in the main clause—about that same thing. So in sentence (1), more knowing means more understanding for the hearer ("you"), and in sentence (2), more size means more falling for whoever "they" are. This kind of coordination happens in English just by putting two clauses together, separated by a comma. It's a concise way of expressing a relationship between two things. Sanskrit allows for a similar kind of expression, using the pair यावत् (*yāvat*) . . . तावत् (*tāvat*). We'll talk more about these kinds of pairings with pronouns in Lesson 8, but for now, we'll treat these two words as *indeclinable*. Indeclinable terms appear in precisely the same form in every context. They don't change according to number, gender, or case.

If we wanted to express example (1) in Sanskrit, instead of repeating "the more," we would replace the first expression with our relative term यावत् (*yāvat*). This co-relates, or pairs with, the correlative term तावत् (*tāvat*). It would be something like:

Example

The more you know, the more you understand.

yāvat you know *tāvat* you understand.

However, usually the *yāvat-tāvat* pair is not translated as "the more . . . the more . . ." but "to the degree that . . . to that same degree" or similarly. That's because we can use this expression for degrees or extents other than a large one ("more"). If we are talking to someone who knows very little, we might use this expression—to the extent that you know, you understand. (Here, what they know and understand isn't much!) So here's how our adaptation of (1) would read in Sanskrit:

Example

*यावत् विन्दसि तावत् बोधसि ।

yāvat vindasi tāvat bodhasi.[2]

2. Pandit point: This sentence would have consonant sandhi applied for the final consonants in the relative-correlative construction: यावद् विन्दसि तावद् बोधसि । *yāvad vindasi*

> To the degree that you learn, in that same degree, you will understand.

Or, extremely concisely:

> You understand what you learn.

Next, we'll look at why verbs like √बुध् (*budh*) become बोधसि (*bodhasi*). (I've given you the first verb, विन्दसि (*vindasi*), in the vocabulary list. Its conjugation pattern is not one we'll learn, but you can look it up in a grammar book—it's a little unusual because of the *nasal infix*, which is the न् (*n*) that appears in the conjugated form.)

7.2.2 Verbs in 8P

> **KEY POINT:** The 8P class has a different stem in the singular than in the dual and plural.

In Lesson 4, we learned a verb that means "to be" or "to exist," √अस् (*as*), which is in 2P, or second class *parasmaipada*. Unlike all of the thematic verbs (1, 4, 6, 10), which have अ (*a*) at the end of their stem form, athematic verbs are different—they don't have अ (*a*) at the end of their stem form. What they *do* have varies. For example, √अस् (*as*), which is 2P, takes endings right onto its root (called a *root stem*). Another athematic class, important for this reading, is 8P, the eighth class. This class has ओ (*o*) and उ (*u*) at the end of the stem. The verb in our reading is an unusual verb form for this class but because it's so common, it's important to learn. It has two different stems, a strong one (करो, *karo-*) and a weak one (कुरु, *kuru-*). The endings are familiar from Lesson 3.

---

tāvad bodhasi. Often, printed Devanāgari editions will not separate at the word boundaries, so it would appear as यावद्विन्दसि तावद्बोधसि ।. See below for more.

Table 37. Present indicative √कृ (*kṛ*) (8P) - to make, to do, to cause

	Singular	Dual	Plural
	strong stem	*weak stem*	
Third person	करोति (*kar**oti***) - he/she/it makes	कुरुतः (*kuru**taḥ***) - those two make	कुर्वन्ति (*kur**vanti***) - they make
Second person	करोषि (*kar**oṣi***) - you make	कुरुथः (*kuru**thaḥ***) - you two make	कुरुथ (*kuru**tha***) - you all make
First person	करोमि (*kar**omi***) - I make	कुर्वः (*kur**vaḥ***) - we two make	कुर्मः (*kur**maḥ***) - we make

The verb √कृ (*kṛ*) changes its meaning when it takes a prefix, as we saw happen with other words in Lesson 5, but it will conjugate the same way. For now, let's leave verbs behind. We'll talk more about them in future lessons.

7.2.3 Sandhi: Word-Final Consonants

> **KEY POINT:** Consonants at the ends of words can change when they encounter vowels at the beginning of another word. Unvoiced and unaspirated consonants become voiced and unaspirated.

You may have noticed that there are a lot of sandhi rules in Sanskrit. One we haven't talked about yet involves consonants at the ends of words. The relative-correlative pair we learned for this lesson is यावत् . . . तावत् (*yāvat . . . tāvat*), and yet the reading has the words यावद् . . . तावन् (*yāvad . . . tāvan*). What's going on? This has to do with voicing in consonants. Below, I've reprinted Table 22 from Lesson 5, which identifies both aspiration and voicing in consonants: consonants with "+" have it, and those with "-" lack it. For instance, the consonants क (*ka*) and त (*ta*) are *unvoiced*. Unvoiced, unaspirated consonants in Sanskrit like these appear at the ends of words, and when they do, they often change to their *voiced* and *unaspirated* counterpart. The counterpart is the consonant in the same row of the table—the consonant articulated in the same place in the mouth. Again, paying attention to how spoken English sounds differ from how we spell them can help you understand this change:

> **Example**
> Printed: "Shut up!"
>
> Spoken: "Shud up!"

This is like how, when the Sanskrit त् (*t*) encounters the vowel उ (*u*), it changes to the voiced equivalent, द् (*d*). See for yourself—saying "Shut up" to someone while enunciating the "t" precisely will take more effort than usual.

Table 22. Consonants in transliteration, with voicing and aspiration

Point of Articulation	Consonants					Semi-Vowels	Sibilants	ह
Voice/aspir.	-V / - A	-V / + A	+V / - A	+V / + A	+V / - A	+V / - A	- V / + A	+V / + A
Guttural	क ka	ख kha	ग ga	घ gha	ङ ṅa			ह ha
Palatal	च ca	छ cha	ज ja	झ jha	ञ ña	य ya	श śa	
Retroflex	ट ṭa	ठ ṭha	ड ḍa	ढ ḍha	ण ṇa	र ra	ष ṣa	
Dental	त ta	थ tha	द da	ध dha	न na	ल la	स sa	
Labial	प pa	फ pha	ब ba	भ bha	म ma	व va		

If you look across the dental row, you might be able to guess why the other change in our reading happens. See Table 38 for two examples of this sandhi pattern.

Table 38. Examples of final consonant sandhi, unvoiced and unaspirated

-V-A Consonant	Initial Sound		+V-A Counterpart	Example
त् (*t*)	nasal	→	न् (n)	*tāvat* + *mitraṃ* → *tāvan* + *mitraṃ* तावत् + मित्रं → तावन्मित्रं (तावन् मित्रं)
त् (*t*)	vowel		द् (d)	*yāvat* + *upakaroti* → *yāvad upakaroti* यावत् + उपकरोति → यावदुप-करोति (यावद् + उपकरोति)

7.3 Putting Everything Together

यावदुपकरोति तावन्मित्रं भवति । उपकारलक्षणं मित्रम् ।

yāvad upakaroti tāvan mitraṃ bhavati. upakāralakṣaṇaṃ mitram.

Our first sentence uses the relative-correlative construction we learned above. To the extent that you've understood the lesson, to that degree, you'll be able to read the first sentence. For a refresher on compounds, turn back to Lesson 2. Remember that Sanskrit verbs do not need an explicit subject. If one is missing, we can match the verb's number and simply insert "one," "he," or "she," depending on context.

Example

ग्रामं गच्छति ।

grāmaṃ gacchati.

One goes to the village.

And don't forget about nominal sentences, way back in Lesson 2. That will help you with the second sentence in the reading, as will thinking about whether a compound is an exocentric compound or a determinative compound.

7.4 About the Reading: Friends and Allies

Before high-powered executives and politicians had books like Stephen R. Covey's *The 7 Habits of Highly Effective People*, Indian rulers and ministers had Kauṭilya's *Arthaśāstra*. It's part of a genre of texts about leadership or good conduct, नीति (*nīti*). Since the book is a compilation of preexisting texts, there is no single date when it was authored. However, in its current form, it probably originated sometime between 175 and 300 CE.[3] Its readers weren't looking for tips on time management but principles for managing a kingdom under an all-powerful monarch who waged wars, levied taxes, and made alliances with other kingdoms. That last topic is what our reading discusses. Allies were so crucial to a kingdom that they are even described as one of its component parts, along with others like the king, the minister, and the land (6.1.1).

Allies, or friends, form part of the "circle of kings" (राजमण्डल, *rāja-maṇḍala*), which we can imagine with the king at the center, and his enemies, allies, enemy's allies, ally's allies, and more extended relationships forming further concentric rings. In some ways, geography was important here: one's nearest territories would be most beneficial as allies. But so is strategy. Knowing whether your neighbors are strong or weak, how their citizens are disposed toward you (if they would be rebellious if you took over), and how your neighbors are related to each other in alliances and conflict are all crucial for savvy ruling. Kauṭilya's text gives principles to help kings navigate these complex sets of conditions.[4]

3. The reasons for these dates, an introduction to the text, and a translation of the entire work are found in Olivelle (2016).

4. See Thapliyal (2021).

The context for our reading is a discussion about what kind of friend or ally is most beneficial to a king. Kauṭilya presents his views in a series of questions, initial (wrong) answers, and then his replies. This formulaic approach is prevalent in Sanskrit texts: the initial view is the पूर्वपक्ष (*pūrvapakṣa*) or position (*pakṣa*) that is earlier (*pūrva*).[5] Our sentence presents Kauṭilya's answer to a question: Which two combinations of features are better in an ally, consistency and non-submissiveness or inconsistency and submissiveness? The पूर्वपक्ष (*pūrvapakṣa*) has said consistency and non-submissiveness are better in an ally. Such an ally might not help you since they don't submit to your desires, but at least they won't hurt you. Kauṭilya rejects this. The inconsistent but submissive ally is better. To see why he thinks so, read the sentence.

5. Pandit point: This is an example of the descriptive compound type that we discussed in Lesson 2.

Lesson 8

Reading: Hitopadeśa 1.39

यस्य मित्रेण सम्भाषो यस्य
मित्रेण संस्थितिः ।
यस्य मित्रेण संलापस्ततो
नास्तीह पुण्यवान् ॥

yasya mitreṇa sambhāṣo yasya mitreṇa
saṃsthitiḥ |
yasya mitreṇa saṃlāpas tato nāstīha
puṇyavān ||

Points of Interest For

The Curious: Focus on the examples to understand 8.2.1; read about the instrumental case in 8.2.3.

The Yoga Aficionado: Two of our vocabulary terms have some meanings in philosophy connected to yoga—look out for a Pandit Point discussing *prakṛti* and *pradhāna*.

The Scholar: After reading, look ahead to Lesson 12 for Sanskrit verse and meter.

8.1 Vocabulary

Devanāgarī	Transliteration	Part of Speech	Translation
इह	iha	indc.	now, here
उपदेश	upadeśa	masc. n.	instruction
ततः	tataḥ	indc.	thus, therefore
तावत्	tāvat	correlative pn.	to the extent that
तृतीया	tṛtīyā	fem. n.	third
पुण्यवान्	puṇyavān	adj., masc. nom. sg.	one who is pious, righteous
प्रकृति	prakṛti	fem. n.	form, pattern
प्रधान	pradhāna	neut. n.	predominant thing; origin
मित्र	mitra	neut. n.	friend
यावत्	yāvat	rel. pn.	to the extent that
लक्षण	lakṣaṇa	neut. n.	characteristic, definition
शोक	śoka	masc. n.	grief, sorrow
श्लोक	śloka	masc. n.	name of a meter; sound, call
सम्भाष	sambhāṣa	masc. n.	conversation, discourse
संलाप	saṃlāpa	masc. n.	conversation, chatter
संस्थिति	saṃsthiti	fem. n.	union, connection
हित	hita	neut. n.	what is appropriate, useful, beneficial
हितोपदेश	hitopadeśa	masc. n., cpd.	*Instruction in What is Appropriate* (title)

8.2 Grammar Notes

KEY POINTS: The relative-correlative construction in Sanskrit allows us to talk about one single thing using different clauses (parts of a sentence that characterize that thing). To track what is being said, it's important to pay attention to gender, case, and number.

Our second reading about friendship comes from a fable told to rascally royals needing an education. This reading is in verse, which is a very common way Sanskrit texts are written, and it is part of the *Hitopadeśa*, or the *Instruction in What is Appropriate*, a collection of stories similar to *Aesop's Fables*, featuring talking animals learning lessons. Within the section on gaining friends (*mitralābha*), we are introduced to the king of the doves, Citragrīva, and the king of the mice, Hiraṇyaka.[1] Citragrīva and his flock have been caught in a net, and he goes to Hiraṇyaka for help, still tangled up in the net's rope. Our verse is one of the lessons from the story, and to understand it, we need to learn more about pronouns.

8.2.1 Relative-Correlative Pairings: Pronouns

KEY POINTS: Relative-correlative constructions are ways to refer to the same thing and describe what it is. Grammatical gender should match between relative and correlative pronouns and between a demonstrative pronoun and its referent. It does not need to match between a noun and its predicate.

We can combine demonstrative pronouns with another kind of pronoun: the relative pronoun. These aren't pronouns you use for your aunts and

1. Pandit point: चित्रग्रीव (*citragrīva*) is an exocentric compound which means "one whose neck (*grīva*) is spotted (*citra*)." हिरण्यक (*hiraṇyaka*) is an adjective which means "one who desires gold."

uncles—they are *relative to* some subject. More precisely, they are relative to a noun in a clause that cannot stand on its own. A "clause" is just a grammatical unit that has a subject and a verb. Some stand on their own as independent clauses. Others depend on, or are *relative to*, these independent clauses. Take the sentence "The turtles ate pizza, which was fresh."

Independent clause

The turtles ate pizza

Relative clause

which was fresh

It is ungrammatical to say "which was fresh" as a complete sentence. It's a relative clause. In other words, the thing it describes that is fresh is *relative to* the independent clause (it's the pizza that's fresh). The relative pronoun in that clause is "which." Relative pronouns in English include "what," "which," "who," "whom," and "that." Note that these aren't the same as the pronouns in questions ("*Which* pizza?" is different than "*which* was pizza").

In Sanskrit, there is one relative pronoun that does all of this work, यद् (*yad*), and it declines like तद् (*tad*).[2] Compare Table 39 below and Table 30 in Lesson 6. You can find the full chart in Appendix 1—just like तद् (*tad*), यद् (*yad*) declines in only seven cases.

2. Pandit point: It's important to note that the Sanskrit relative pronoun does not play the role of "who" or "what" in *questions*. There is a special pronoun for that, which we'll see in Lesson 10. But once you know the declension for the demonstrative pronoun, you also know it for the relative and interrogative pronoun! While सः (*saḥ*) is the masculine demonstrative pronoun "he" or "that," and यः (*yaḥ*) is the relative pronoun "who," the interrogative pronoun is कः (*kaḥ*) and—that's right—it declines like the masculine pronoun तद् (*tad*).

Table 39. Relative pronoun, masculine, nominative (यद्/*yad*)

	Singular	Dual	Plural
Nominative	यः **yaḥ** (that which)	यौ **yau** (those two which)	ये **ye** (those which)

While the relative pronoun does the same thing as "which" in our English sentence above (it refers to a noun in an independent clause), it doesn't do it in the same order. In Sanskrit, the order of the sentence would be different. The relative pronoun comes first:

Example
Which (*yad*) pizza was fresh, **that (*tad*)** the turtles ate.

Relative pronouns are almost always found paired with demonstrative pronouns, as we'll see next.

One benefit to learning Sanskrit grammar is that it draws our attention to grammar in ordinary cases. For instance, the American singer-songwriter Christina Aguilera has lyrics that, while not as profound, use the same grammatical structure as the *Chāndogya Upaniṣad*: a relative-correlative construction. This sentence structure indicates that the *same thing* is being talked about in two phrases. In Aguilera's lyrics, the single thing being talked about is the person she's singing to, a "somebody" who is sensitive, courageous, etc. It is that same person who is referred to by "*What* a girl wants" and "*What* a girl needs." To appreciate the syntax, let's rewrite the sentence by making the implied "is" explicit and focusing on just one of the things that (Aguilera thinks) a girl wants.

Example
What a girl wants is somebody sensitive.

Here, the pronoun "what" refers to the same thing as the pronoun "somebody." These pronouns are *coordinated*. Let's look at an example of such coordination in Sanskrit. We'll go back to our vocabulary from Lesson 2 when we learned the definition of yoga: योगश्चित्तवृत्तिनिरोधः (*yogaś cittavṛttinirodhaḥ*). This sentence tells us that yoga is the cessation of mental activity. We can put this in a relative-correlative form in English using the *yad-tad* form:

Example

That which (*yad*) is yoga, **that (*tad*)** is the cessation of mental activity.

In Sanskrit, the sentence would be:

Example (without sandhi)

*यः योगः सः चित्तवृत्तिनिरोधः अस्ति ।

*yaḥ yogaḥ saḥ cittavṛttinirodhaḥ asti.

Example (with sandhi)

यो योगः सश्चित्तवृत्तिनिरोधो ऽस्ति ।

yo yogaḥ saścittavṛttinirodho 'sti.

As we've learned, the verb is optional—we could just write the sentence with the pair of pronouns. The pairing of relative and correlative pronouns is so common that you'll hear Sanskritists talk about this as a *yad-tad* construction. Since word order is fairly free, don't always expect the *yad* to come first—though it usually does—in the reverse of how we typically speak in English.

Sanskrit relative-correlative constructions are very useful because they can compactly refer to previous terms. Due to grammatical gender and number, it's easy to distinguish between "this" and "that" in Sanskrit since the gender and numbers of pronouns and their referents must match, as we've already seen (go back to Lesson 6 for a refresher). Likewise, relative-correlative constructions must match. Since योगः (*yogaḥ*) is masculine nominative singular, the pronouns referring to it must be यः (*yaḥ*) and सः (*saḥ*).

What's important in reading these complex sentences (and really, any sentences with pronouns) is to keep an eye on the grammatical gender, number, and case. For instance, here's how a Sanskrit adaptation of Christina Aguilera's lyrics might go:

Example

Original:

What a girl wants is somebody sensitive and courageous.

Relative-correlative form:

That which a girl wants is that one who is a sensitive person and brave person.

Sanskrit (without sandhi):

*यम् कन्या इच्छति सः सहृदयः वीरः च ।

yam kanyā icchati saḥ sahṛdayaḥ vīraḥ ca.

That which (*yam*) a girl (*kanyā*) wants (*icchati*) is that one who is (*saḥ*) a sensitive person (*sahṛdayaḥ*) and (*ca*) brave person (*viraḥ*).

Sanskrit (with sandhi):

यं कन्येच्छति स सहृदयो वीरश्च ।

yaṃ kanyecchati sa sahṛdayo vīraś ca.

8.2.2 Conjunctions, च (*ca*) and वा (*vā*)

KEY POINT: Sanskrit conjunctions appear between words and at the end of a series of words.

You might wonder why the word for "and," च (*ca*), is all the way at the end in that last sentence instead of between सहृदयः (*sahṛdayaḥ*) and वीरः (*vīraḥ*). That's because *conjunctions* in Sanskrit often appear at the end of two paired words:

Pattern

word1 and word2

word1 word2 च

Example

*सहृदयः वीरः च → सहृदयो वीरश्च

*sahṛdayaḥ vīraḥ ca → sahṛdayo vīraś ca

sensitive and courageous

When there are a lot of words conjoined, you may see the indeclinable conjunction between each of them and then again at the end:

Pattern

word1 and word2 and word3 and word4

word1 च word2 च word3 च word4 च

Example

*धर्मः च कामः च अर्थः च मोक्षः च → धर्मश्च कामश्चार्थश्च मोक्षश्च

*dharmaḥ ca kāmaḥ ca arthaḥ ca mokṣaḥ ca → dharmaś ca kāmaś ca arthaś ca mokṣaś ca

duty and desire and wealth and liberation

You'll need to keep an eye out for sibilant sandhi with the conjunction. Finally, the word for disjunction, "or," is वा (*vā*), and it works the same way as च (*ca*), in that it can appear at the end of a pair or, for a series, between each word and again at the end.

8.2.3 More about the Instrumental Case

KEY POINT: The instrumental case conveys how some action happens, like the English preposition "by" or "with."

Our third grammar section is, appropriately, about the *instrumental*. Why appropriately? Because in the traditional list of cases, the instrumental is third and is known in Sanskrit by that name, तृतीया (*tṛtīyā*). A noun in the instrumental case is roughly equivalent to a noun that has the English preposition "by" or "with" before it. Using this case marks the object as an instrument, method, or means (see 10.2.5 for another use, the passive construction).

For instance, suppose I wanted to say that we use योग (*yoga*) to engage in the cessation of mental activity (as we learned in Lesson 2). Since it is the *way* that I perform this cessation, I might say:

Example

Cessation of mental activity is *by yoga*.

As we learned in Lesson 3, rather than adding "by," I add an ending to योग (*yoga*). It becomes योगेन (*yogena*). This is the form for the singular instrumental. Just as with our other cases, we can form the instrumental in the dual and the plural, as Table 40 shows. Other masculine and neuter nouns which end in अ (*a*) will follow the same pattern.

Table 40. *a*-stem masculine, instrumental (योग/*yoga*)

	Singular	Dual	Plural
Instrumental (means)	योगेन (yogena) – by yoga	योगाभ्याम् (yogābhyām) – by the two yogas	योगैः (yogaiḥ) – by the many yogas

Nouns in the instrumental case relate to verbs, whether explicit or implied. Often, the instrumental case expresses the *means* by which some action occurs. We can illustrate this with the sentence above:

Example

योगेन चित्तवृत्तिनिरोधो ऽस्ति । yogena cittavṛttinirodho 'sti.

Cessation of mental activity (*cittavṛttinirodhaḥ*)[3] is (*asti*) by yoga (*yogena*).

3. Don't forget your *visarga* sandhi! If you're not sure where the ओ (*o*) came from, go back to Lesson 5.

Or, since Sanskrit often uses nominal sentences, we could drop the verb and just say:

Example
योगेन चित्तवृत्तिनिरोधः । yogena cittavṛttinirodhaḥ.

Cessation of mental activity (*cittavṛttinirodhaḥ*) [is] by yoga (*yogena*).

Both of these sentences express that the occurring, or the coming into existence, of चित्तवृत्तिनिरोधः (*cittavṛttinirodhaḥ*) is by means of योग (*yoga*).

Another use for the instrumental is to express the idea of *accompanying*. This is different. If I go to the restaurant *with my friends*, I'm not going in the same way as when I go to the restaurant *by bus*. My friends accompany my action. They aren't the instrument that carries out my action:

Example
मित्रेण रामो गच्छति ।

mitreṇa[4] rāmo gacchati.

Rāma goes *with* a friend.[5]

This sense of the instrumental also occurs even without an explicit verb when the action of possession is implied:

Example
मित्रेण रामस्य सम्भाषः।

mitreṇa rāmasya sambhāṣaḥ.

A conversation of Rāma is with a friend.

Or: Rāma has conversation *with* a friend.

---

4. Why is there a ण (*ṇa*) at the end of this word? Go back to Lesson 5 to remind yourself.

5. Pandit point: Often, the adverb सह (*saha*), equivalent to "with," comes directly after the instrumental: मित्रेण सह रामो गच्छति । *mitreṇa saha rāmo gacchati*, "Rama goes with a friend."

Remember that the genitive conveys possession. And that's more naturally expressed in English as "Rāma has conversation" than "of Rama there is conversation." Also, remember that our usual word order in Sanskrit is subject, object (or predicate), verb. When additional nouns are inserted into the sentence, they are typically close to the words they modify, but not always, especially in verse.

8.2.4 Feminine Nouns: *i*-stem

KEY POINT: Feminine nouns ending in an *i*-stem are very common, and the table in this section is useful to learn (or bookmark).

One of the nouns in your reading is in a new declension pattern: संस्थिति (*saṃsthiti*). To help you learn the form, a new vocabulary word below illustrates the pattern. It's also a common term that means "pattern" or "form."[6]

Table 41. *i*-stem feminine, nominative (प्रकृति/*prakṛti*)

	Singular	Dual	Plural
Nominative	प्रकृतिः prakṛti**ḥ** (a pattern)	प्रकृती prakṛt**ī** (two patterns)	प्रकृतयः prakṛt**ayaḥ** (many patterns)

An important reminder about grammatical gender: while it needs to match for adjectives and nouns, it doesn't for nominal sentences. This

6. Pandit point: The words प्रकृतिः (*prakṛtiḥ*) and प्रधानम् (*pradhānam*) are also important words in Indian philosophy, with some further meanings. While *prakṛtiḥ* can just mean "pattern," for Sāṃkhya (a philosophical tradition whose name means "enumeration"), the term refers to the original material stuff out of which everything has come to exist. In this way, the cosmological pattern is the origin, the *pradhāna*. In Mīmāṃsā (meaning, "desire to know"), a tradition focused on understanding Vedic rituals, the *prakṛti* is an important ritual that is the pattern for other rituals (and which may be adapted slightly). Plenty of other uses for these terms and more nuanced connotations exist in different contexts.

means I can talk about something or someone's having a form using a masculine or neuter pronoun:

Example

प्रकृतिः प्रधानम् ।

prakṛtiḥ pradhānam.

The pattern is the origin.

However, the relative-correlative pair should match in gender:

Example

यस्य प्रकृतिः सो भवति ।

yasya prakṛtiḥ so bhavati.

Of that which has a pattern, it exists.

Or: What has a pattern exists.

8.2.5 Introduction to Sanskrit Verse

> **KEY POINT:** Verse is a common way Sanskrit is written, and understanding short and long vowels is crucial for reading it.

This lesson's reading is in verse. One reason we can tell is that the first line ends in a single *daṇḍa* (।) and the second in a double *daṇḍa* (॥). Here, single *daṇḍa* isn't a period. It's a pause that divides the verse into halves. Quite a lot of Sanskrit literature is written in verse form, although, unlike English verse, where you might expect a lot of rhyming, Sanskrit verse depends on alternations of light and heavy syllables. A syllable is made up either of a single vowel or a consonant followed by a vowel. Our vocab term √भू (*bhū*) is a single syllable, while योग (*yoga*) is made up of two: यो.ग (*yo.ga*)—the period shows the syllable division. The difference between short and long vowels that we learned in Lesson 4 is important here: when a syllable ends with a short vowel, it's light, and when it ends with a long vowel or a diphthong like ओ (*o*), it's heavy.

A short vowel is counted as long when it's followed by two consonants. (The visarga and anusvāra count as consonants.)

Both for our reading and others like it, being in a metrical form made it easier to memorize. Each meter has its own name, and one of the most common is the श्लोक (*śloka*), the meter in this lesson. Tradition has it that the famous poet Vālmīki was spontaneously inspired to create this meter when he heard the plaintive cries of a bird who had lost its mate. This cry of grief, or शोक (*śoka*), gave rise to what he called the श्लोक (*śloka*). Although our reading is ordered very much like a prose sentence, word order in Sanskrit verse can be fairly free since the verb conjugations and noun declensions tell us what role each word plays. This can make reading Sanskrit in verse more challenging than prose. For more detail on verse, see Lesson 12.

8.3 Putting Everything Together

यस्य मित्रेण सम्भाषो यस्य मित्रेण संस्थितिः ।

यस्य मित्रेण संलापस्ततो नास्तीह पुण्यवान् ॥

yasya mitreṇa sambhāṣo yasya mitreṇa saṃsthitiḥ |

yasya mitreṇa saṃlāpas tato nāstīha puṇyavān ||

Don't forget to look for sandhi as you read this verse. Remember our slippery *visarga*, which transforms into sibilants sometimes. And don't forget the principles of vowel combinations we learned in Lesson 4.

You should also remind yourself of the genitive case from Lesson 5. Remember that the English word "of," which is how the genitive is often translated, has a range of meanings. It's important to be clear in what sense you understand it. A team *of* turtles is a team that is composed by turtles. But a box *of* pizza contains pizza; it isn't composed by pizza. And the king *of* England does not contain England, but England belongs to him—he possesses it.

Another tip for reading this verse is to find the main verb first. Despite the single *daṇḍa* at the end of the first line, we treat the two lines together as an entire sentence. And, as we've learned, verbs usually come toward the end of sentences. Finally, another helpful trick is to find clauses and treat them in groups. There is no better Sanskrit student than one who reads with patience, one who breaks sandhi with patience, one who analyzes verses with patience.

8.4 About the Reading: Friends, Allies, and Governance

Friendship is crucial for ruling a kingdom, as we saw in the last lesson—kings need to make allies with neighboring kingdoms. Our young princes need to learn not only how to make alliances, but also how to navigate relationships within courtly life. In this story, even though the the animals are kings who become allies, their relationships might illustrate lessons about friendships. Ministers within a single king's court also must form friendships and alliances.[7]

At the beginning of the lesson, we left Citragrīva ensnared in a net with his flock, heading to Hiraṇyaka for help. The king of the mice is said to know the science of leadership, नीतिशास्त्र (*nītiśāstra*), and he's holed up deep in his nest, concerned about crows who might come to eat him and his mousy subjects. Although initially quiet when Citragrīva arrives and calls out, the mouse king recognizes his poor winged friend and comes out, saying how happy he is to see him. Then King Hiraṇyaka recites our lesson's verse, which suggests there's more than just political expediency in their relationship. However, we shouldn't mistake their friendship as being entirely removed from the pragmatic questions of

7. For different interpretations of this story and its relationship to the *Arthaśāstra*, see Patil (2017).

governance.[8] Eventually, after some discussion of who should be cut free first—Citragrīva argues that Hiraṇyaka should free his dove subjects first, not himself—the mouse gnaws the ropes apart.

However, this isn't the end of the section on gaining friends! A crow has been watching the events and swoops down, proposing friendship with the mice and the doves. Hiraṇyaka is skeptical and explains his concerns with a story (there are several layers of stories within stories in the *Hitopadeśa*). I won't spoil the ending for you. If you continue on with Sanskrit, you can read this text in Charles Lanman's *Sanskrit Reader*, which is freely available online because it is out of copyright.

8. The term मित्र (*mitra*) in this context seems to include both personal/private and formal/public relationships together. For discussion, see Ali (2004, 183–84).

Lesson 9

Reading: Mahābhārata 5.34.10

न राज्यं प्राप्तमित्येव
वर्तितव्यमसांप्रतम् ।
श्रियं ह्यविनयो हन्ति जरा
रूपमिवोत्तमम् ॥

na rājyaṃ prāptam ity eva vartitavyam
asāṃpratam |
śriyaṃ hy avinayo hanti jarā rūpam
ivottamam ||

Points of Interest For

The Curious: As this lesson includes a longer reading that builds on previous material, you might want to look at 9.3 Putting Everything Together first and work your way through each of the four parts of the reading discussed there.

The Yoga Aficionado: This lesson will explain (sort of) how the Buddha got his name, in the discussion of past passive participles.

The Scholar: The material on comparison in 9.2.4 will be relevant for Lesson 12's discussion of Sanskrit poetry.

9.1 Vocabulary

Devanāgarī	Transliteration	Part of Speech	Translation
√आप् (+प्र)	√āp (+ pra)	v. (5P)	attained, acquired, reached
इव	iva	indc.	like, as if
उत्तम	uttama	adj.	highest; best
एव	eva	ind.	indeed, really, truly
कन्या	kanyā	fem. n.	girl, young woman
जरा	jarā	fem. n.	old age
नित्य	nitya	adj.	eternal, permanent
पद्म	padma	neut. n.	lotus
प्राप्त	prāpta	ppp.	has been acquired
भारत	bhārata	masc. n.	descendants of Bharata
महत्	mahat	adj.	great
मुख	mukha	neut. n.	face, mouth
√राज्	√rāj	v. (1P)	rule, govern
राज्य	rājya	neut. n.	kingdom
रूप	rūpa	neut. n.	beauty; physical form
विनय	vinaya	masc. n.	discipline, restraint
√वृत्	√vṛt	v. (1A)	engaged in, done, employed
श्री	śrī	fem. n.	name of Lakṣmī; prosperity, wealth, success

सांप्रतम्	sāṃpratam	indc. (adv.)	appropriately, suitably
√हन्	han	v. (2P)	destroy, kill
हन्ति	hanti	3 sg. √*han* (2P)	he/she/it destroys
हि	hi	indc.	for, because

9.2 Grammar Notes

KEY POINTS: Adjectives in Sanskrit work similarly to nouns, as they are case declined. This lesson also introduces you to verbal adjectives—which are also case declined.

The reading for this lesson comes from one of the longest epics ever written, the *Mahābhārata*, about the violent and dramatic challenges facing the Bhārata dynasty's succession. It has intrigue, battles, magic, and family feuds and is more than 200,000 verses long. It's also the source of the famous *Bhagavadgītā*, one of the most translated books ever, probably second only to the Bible. Like the *Hitopadeśa*, the *Mahābhārata* is primarily written in the verse form *śloka*, which we learned about in Lesson 8. However, the word order in this lesson is close to prose patterns, which helps introduce us to the relationship between finite verbs and other kinds of verbal forms. Finite verbs aren't contrasted with *in*finite verbs, but *non*-finite verbs (a good thing if you ever want to finish this book). While non-finite verbs—like the verbs we've already learned—follow regular patterns and are derived from verb roots, they act like adjectives.

9.2.1 Adjectives

KEY POINT: Adjectives in Sanskrit match the gender, number, and case of the noun they modify.

Adjectives modify nouns—they're descriptive words. In Sanskrit, like in English, adjectives usually come before the noun that they modify:

Pattern

adjective noun

Example

उत्तम आत्मा

uttama ātmā

highest self

In this example, उत्तम (*uttama*) is declined like योगः (*yogaḥ*) in the masculine nominative singular. (The *visarga* has disappeared because of sandhi.) That's because it follows the *a*-stem declension, as we learned in Lesson 3. We don't need to learn new declensions specific to adjectives. All we need to do is pay attention to the ending of the word in its stem form in the dictionary.[1] That tells us which declension pattern it uses. For example, you'll notice the ending of उत्तम (*uttama*) isn't the same as the ending for आत्मा (*ātmā*). That's because the noun आत्मा (*ātmā*) declines differently than उत्तम (*uttama*): it's an *an*-stem, as we will learn in Lesson 10. You can add many adjectives before a noun, and you'll know which noun they modify by recognizing their endings:

Pattern

adjective adjective noun

Example

नित्य उत्तम आत्मा

nitya uttama ātmā

eternal highest self

1. Pandit point: The categories of nouns and adjectives, so familiar to English grammar students, aren't found in Sanskrit grammars. Traditional Sanskrit grammars distinguish between नाम (*nāma*) and आख्यात (*ākhyāta*)—nominals and action words. What we'd call "adjectives" would fall under नाम (*nāma*), which most people translate as "noun," whereas आख्यात (*ākhyāta*) is typically translated as "verb."

This is why, when you learn adjectives, it's important to understand their declension patterns. Both उत्तम (*uttama*) and नित्य (*nitya*), because they are *a*-stems, will follow that declension pattern when modifying a noun if the noun is masculine or neuter. For the most part, when modifying feminine nouns, *a*-stem adjectives will follow the *ā*-stem declension (Table 42). Some will follow the declension for *prakṛti* instead (see Table 41 in Lesson 8 or check Appendix 1), and some have an option between the two. We've seen parts of the first two declensions already. Also, notice that there is no vowel sandhi between नित्य (*nitya*) and उत्तम (*uttama*). Sandhi changes only happen once. We don't keep combining sounds. Since the two vowels are not combined into a diphthong, we know there was an earlier change. Compare:

Visarga sandhi

Original
*नित्यः उत्तमः आत्मा
**nityaḥ uttamaḥ ātmā*

Sandhi applied
नित्य उत्तम आत्मा
nitya uttama ātmā

Vowel sandhi

Original
*नित्य उत्तम आत्मा
**nitya uttama ātmā*

Sandhi applied
नित्योत्तमात्मा
nityottamātmā

In the second example, either we have adjectives that do not modify the noun since they don't match the case, or we have a compound. Quick self-test: If this were not a compound, what case would नित्य (*nitya*) and उत्तम (*uttama*) be? If you don't remember, check your *a*-stem declension chart.

For grammatically feminine words, the declension pattern is not an *a*-stem, but an *ā*-stem.

Table 42. *ā*-stem feminine, nominative/ accusative (कन्या/*kanyā*)

	Singular	Dual	Plural
Nominative (subject)	कन्या (kany**ā**) – a girl	कन्ये (kany**e**) – two girls	कन्याः (kany**āḥ**) – many girls
Accusative (object)	कन्याम् (kany**ām**) – a girl	कन्ये (kany**e**) – two girls	कन्याः (kany**āḥ**) – many girls

An a-stem adjective would decline like this when modifying a feminine noun. We'd just apply the endings in bold. With this in mind, here's how *uttama* would appear modifying different nouns (notice the sandhi!):

Adjective noun

उत्तमा कन्या
uttamā kanyā
excellent young woman

उत्तमं सुत्रम्
uttamaṃ sūtram
excellent *sūtra*

उत्तमो देवः
uttamo devaḥ
excellent (or "highest") god

Finally, a note about translating adjectives: There are different shades of meaning to all words, depending on how they're used, but this fact is especially important with adjectives. We might translate the same word differently depending on what the adjective modifies. (Compare the "Great Lakes" to a "great day." What synonyms could you use to distinguish the two meanings of "great"?)

9.2.2 Past Passive Participles

KEY POINT: Past passive participles add -त (*-ta*) to the end of a verb root to convey an action was performed.

Now I'll explain *exciting* participles, those *anticipated* participles you have been *waiting* for! That sentence includes two participles: *exciting* and *anticipated*. These are participles because they are formed from verbs (excite, anticipate) and act as modifiers or part of a verb phrase. And even though "waiting" is not modifying a noun, it is a predicate– it's what you have been doing. In Sanskrit, participles decline to match the nouns they modify (and their predicates). That's why they're often called *verbal adjectives*. One of the most common is the *past passive participle*, which expresses an activity that was done in the past. That it's passive means that the action was done to something by some other agent. You can use the zombie test to see that a verb (or participle) is passive. Add "by zombies" after the verb in question. If it makes sense, it's passive. For example:

> The kingdom was acquired *by zombies*.[2]

Here, "was acquired" is a past passive participle. To form this in English, we add -ed and the helping verb "was." In Sanskrit, we (often) simply add -त (*-ta*) to the end of a verb root:

Pattern
root + ta = past passive participle

---

2. In Lesson 10, we'll see how we could write this in Sanskrit using the instrumental: राज्यं प्राप्तं वेतालाभिः (*rājyaṃ prāptaṃ vetālābhiḥ*). A *vetāla* isn't exactly one of George A. Romero's zombies but a spirit called forth by Tantric practitioners to possess dead bodies in cremation grounds. See Huang (2009).

Example

prāp + ta = prāpta

प्राप् + त = प्राप्त

With the verbs we've seen earlier, we can do the same thing:

√भू + त = भूत *bhūta*, "was" or "has occurred"
√कृ + त = कृत *kṛta*, "was done" or "was made"
√बुध् + त = बुद्ध *buddha*,[3] "was enlightened" or "the Buddha"
√विद् + इ + त = विदित *vidita*, "was known" or "was learned"

Notice the last verb needs a vowel, इ (*i*), in between the root and the ending for us to be able to pronounce it, but we don't add this vowel to the root of √बुध् (*budh*). You'll learn these patterns by experience—there isn't an easy way to anticipate all of them. (You can also look up verb roots in Whitney's *The Roots, Verb-Forms, and Primary Derivatives of the Sanskrit Language*.) Past passive participles—or "PPP"s, for short—have a few uses.

Verbal

Instead of a finite verb, we can use a PPP.

Example

राज्यं **प्राप्तम्**

rājyaṃ ***prāptam*.**

The kingdom **has been acquired.**

---

3. Pandit point: Sandhi strikes again! This change, from the aspirated ध् (*-dh*) to the consonant conjunct -द्ध (*-ddha*) is very common. (Here's the conjunct again, larger: द्ध) It's because aspirating naturally comes after the consonant conjunct and shifting from a voiced consonant to an unvoiced is also hard. Try to say "budh-ta" with the aspiration only after the first consonant and without any voicing in the second. It's tough. So, the aspiration moves to the second syllable, and the second consonant also becomes voiced. Given this pattern, try to predict the past passive participle of √युध् (*yudh*).

In this example, the agent—the one who acquired the kingdom—is missing. Is it zombies? Soldiers? We don't know. But it is a complete sentence.

Adjectival

Another way ppp's are used is as adjectives. These are best translated in English using relative clauses (see Lesson 7). For instance, the phrase

Example

राज्यं **प्राप्तम्**

rājyaṃ ***prāptam***

. . . kingdom **that has been acquired** . . .

might be found in a longer sentence:

Example

मित्रं **राज्यं प्राप्तं** हन्ति ।

mitraṃ ***rājyaṃ prāptam*** *hanti.*

The ally destroys the **kingdom that has been acquired**.

To determine whether the participle is acting as an adjective or a noun, we must pay attention to context and whether there are other finite verbs in the sentence.

Substantival

You've already seen past passive participles in this role, where they have disguised themselves as nouns. This is a *substantival* use of a participle and you saw it in our second lesson:

Example

चित् + त = चित्त

cit + ta = citta

what was thought, a thought

In context, the participle acts as a noun, "thought." It is embedded within a compound in that reading, चित्तवृत्तिनिरोध (*cittavṛttinirodha*), "cessation of the activity of thought." The word does not act as an adjective: the activity is not something that has been thought. Because they are like nouns, these substantival uses will need a verb (implicit or explicit) to make them into a complete sentence. Often, you can look up PPPs in a dictionary and find their own entry. The word प्राप्त (*prāpta*), for instance, can mean "achievement," something "which has been acquired"; it can also be used for a person, "someone who has achieved," whether that achievement is material or spiritual. In all the examples above, the PPP will decline to match the noun. In the masculine or neuter, it will follow the *a*-stem pattern we've learned; in the feminine, typically the *ā*-stem, as mentioned above.

9.2.3 Future Passive Participles (Gerundives)

> **KEY POINT:** Future passive participles add -तव्य or -य (*-tavya* or *-ya*) to the end of a verb stem to convey an action must or needs to be performed.

Now, we are getting into a concept that simply *must be learned*. It *has to be understood*, even though there is no strictly analogous grammatical feature in English. Both "must be learned" and "has to be understood" are ways to translate the gerundive, also known as a future passive participle. In our reading, वर्तितव्यम् (*vartitavyam*) is an example of a gerundive, derived from the 1A verb √वृत् (*vṛt*). This is another participle that declines to modify a noun. These participles have the force of something that *should* or *must* happen, not just something that *will* happen. These are recognizable by their तव्य (*-tavya*) ending, although some will only have a य (*-ya*) ending.[4] Grammar books like Whitney's *Roots, Verb-Forms, and Primary Derivatives* will help you identify which

---

4. Pandit point: The word राज्य (*rājya*), which means "kingdom," is a gerundive with this ending. That's because a kingdom is something that must be ruled, from the 1P verb

verbs have which endings and how their roots transform. In this case, there is a strengthening from वृत् (*vṛt*) to वर्त् (*vart*), and then an intermediate इ (*i*) is inserted, not unlike we saw above in विदित (*vidita*).

Pattern

verb stem (+ *i*) + *tavya* (or -*ya*) + ending

Example

(वृत् + strengthening) + इ + तव्य + म् = वर्तितव्यम्

(*vṛt* + strengthening) + *i* + *tavya* + *m* = *vartitavyam*

The appropriate case ending for the noun in our reading is neuter, nominative, singular. All masculine and neuter gerundives decline following the *a*-stem pattern. Feminine gerundives follow the *ā*-stem pattern.

9.2.4 Comparisons

KEY POINT: The indeclinable word इव (*iva*) expresses similarity between two things.

Our reading includes a comparison word: इव (*iva*), which can be translated as "like" or "as." Sanskrit has a long poetic tradition that makes extensive use of comparisons—see Lesson 12. Faces are like moons, and eyes are like lotuses. Our example comparison includes a noun phrase (an adjective and a noun together) and a noun, but verbs can also be the subject of comparison. The pattern is simple:

Pattern

x इव y

x *iva* y

y is like x

√राज् (*rāj*). However, you would not translate the word in our reading as "what must be ruled"! This is why context is crucial.

Like our quotative particle इति (*iti*), this indeclinable is a postposition, which means it appears after the word it modifies. This is important since it means that the target of the comparison is *x* in the pattern above:

Example

*पद्मम् इव मुखम् ।

पद्ममिव मुखम् ।[5]

padmam iva mukham.

The face (*mukham*) is like a lotus (*padmam*).

Order is important. Someone's face being like a lotus is different than a lotus floating in a pond that looks like a human face! We can add adjectives, too:

Example

भद्रं पद्ममिव मुखम् ।

bhadraṃ padmam iva mukham.

The face is like a beautiful lotus.

Of course, as with any Sanskrit word, it's imperative to keep an eye out for sandhi, as this small word can easily become combined with others, and you might miss it.

9.2.5 Indeclinables: एव (*eva*), हि (*hi*)

> **KEY POINT:** एव (*eva*) intensifies the word that precedes it, and हि (*hi*) expresses a reason. Both are indeclinable terms.

This reading introduces you to two more important indeclinable terms. The first, एव (*eva*), is known as an *intensifier*. This means that it makes

5. If you don't remember why the final म् (*-m*) and the initial इ (*i*) conjoin in the Devanāgarī and not the transliteration, go back to Lesson 6.

another meaning more intense. Its intensifying powers focus on the prior word, which I illustrate by underlining and italicizing the words in the sample pattern:

Pattern

blah *blah* एव

Precisely what this intensification amounts to depends on context. Sometimes, it means "only"; other times, it means "indeed," "truly," or, in a concessive sense, "even."

Example

अहं धर्मं करोमि ।

ahaṃ dharmaṃ karomi.

I engage in *dharma*. (= I perform/do *dharma*)

Notice how the position of the word changes the meaning:

अहमेव धर्मं करोमि ।
aham eva dharmaṃ karomi.
I alone engage in *dharma*. (= I'm the only person who performs/does *dharma*.)
अहं धर्ममेव करोमि ।
ahaṃ dharmam eva karomi.
I engage in *dharma* alone. (= I perform/do only *dharma*, nothing else.)

When it comes after the quotative marker इति (*iti*), the intensifier operates on the whole thing that has been said. It stresses the utterance.

Example

अहं धर्मं करोमीति वदति ।
ahaṃ dharmaṃ karomīti vadati.
"I engage in *dharma*," he says.

अहं धर्मं करोमीत्येव वदति ।
ahaṃ dharmaṃ karomīty eva vadati.
"I engage in *dharma*," he even says. (= Doubting what he says)
"I engage in *dharma*," he says, truly. (= Emphasizing what he says)
He says only, "I engage in *dharma*." (= He says nothing else.)

Context is essential for understanding this particle. If the speaker is someone who frequently lies, we might interpret the particle as "even" (can you believe he said that?).

The other particle in our reading, हि (*hi*), usually means "because" and is found at the start of a clause giving a reason. You won't see it at the very beginning of a sentence, but it will come after the first word:

Pattern
अहं हि धर्मं करोमि ।

ahaṃ hi dharmaṃ karomi.

Because I engage in *dharma*.[6]

9.2.6 Adverbs

KEY POINT: Adverbs communicate how an action happens, and you recognize adverbs in Sanskrit based on their role, not their form.

Another kind of word that is indeclinable in Sanskrit is the *adverb*. An adverb expresses how an action is performed. Is the killing performed *softly*, as the Fugees describe the impact of a singer's words, or is it performed *harshly, brutally, kindly, quickly* . . . ? English tends to use -ly

6. Pandit point: Yes, you can start a sentence with the word "because" in English. And you can start a sentence with any conjunction—there is nothing ungrammatical about it. It's a matter of style.

to indicate that a word is an adverb. Sanskrit, in contrast, doesn't distinguish adverbs by their form (their morphology). Instead, we must determine whether a word in question is modifying a noun (in which case it could be an adjective) or a verb (in which case it could be an adverb). In our reading, the word असांप्रतम् (*asāṃpratam*) is an adverb since it modifies the past passive participle. It tells us how the kingdom has been acquired and in what manner.[7]

9.3 Putting Everything Together

न राज्यं प्राप्तमित्येव वर्तितव्यमसांप्रतम् ।
श्रियं ह्यविनयो हन्ति जरा रूपमिवोत्तमम् ॥

na rājyaṃ prāptam ity eva vartitavyam asāṃpratam |
śriyaṃ hy avinayo hanti jarā rūpam ivottamam ||

When you compare the printed Devanāgarī with the transliteration, you'll see that several of the words are printed together in Devanāgarī, as we've learned about in 6.2.3. If you have a hard time reading the Devanāgarī, start with the transliteration and look back. When you encounter words printed together in Devanāgarī but not in the transliteration, remember why and look for any sandhi that may have happened.

While not a hard-and-fast rule, one useful heuristic for reading verses is to look for syntactical units that correspond to the four quarters:

7. Pandit point: Just what counts as an "adverb" in Sanskrit is surprisingly controversial. You will find different opinions among lexicographers (the authors of dictionaries) and, like with adjectives and nouns, Sanskrit grammarians themselves don't seem to have considered them a unified category. See Gombrich (1979) for a discussion of the topic and Ajotikar and Kulkarni (2016) for a survey of various dictionaries and grammars in the context of applications in computer programming known as Natural Language Processing.

1. na rājyaṃ prāptam ity eva
2. vartitavyam asāṃpratam
3. śriyaṃ hy avinayo hanti
4. jarā rūpam ivottamam.

Starting with the first quarter, it's necessary to recognize that the *iti*-clause expresses something a person has said or thought. There's no explicit verb for saying or thinking, but we can insert one in our translation:

Saying/thinking "*rājyaṃ prāptam*" . . .

The second quarter includes a gerundive (future passive participle), वर्तितव्यम् (*vartitavyam*), which is negated with the verse's initial न (*na*). A hint: you might initially think the gerundive is part of the *iti*-clause, but when you read the entire verse, that interpretation doesn't make as much sense. Instead, this gerundive modifies असांप्रतम् (*asāṃpratam*) as a verbal adjective. Remember that we've learned how negations and the verb they negate can be separated by several words.

Our third quarter gives a reason for what has come before, with our particle हि (*hi*) and a present indicative verb, हन्ति (*hanti*). Although this verb form might look like the plural, it is formed following the pattern we saw with the 2P verb √अस् (*as*). And the ending -ति (*-ti*) is added directly to हन् (*han*), as it is a root stem verb. Go back to Lesson 4 for a refresher on the 2P form. Your case endings will help you identify what is the subject and object of this verb.

Finally, the fourth quarter involves a comparison. The verb in the third quarter is implicitly part of this comparison: *x* verbs *y* like *a* (verbs) *b*. In English, we usually have the verb in both parts of the comparison since it doesn't make sense syntactically otherwise. English doesn't usually say: "A woman needs a man like a fish a bicycle." Sanskrit does. In this last quarter, keep an eye out for adjectives, too.

Once you've read through the verse and gotten a sense of the four main units of meaning, see if you can put it all together into a single sentence describing what should not be the case and why.

9.4 About the Reading: Good Advice

This lesson's reading is a two-in-one. That's because it's found in both the *Hitopadeśa* and the *Mahābhārata*. But the *Mahābhārata* is much older, and the *Hitopadeśa* is quoting from it. This quotation comes from a section known as the "Preparations" (*udyoga*) section, where the preparations are for war between the Pāṇḍava and the Kaurava families. In a nutshell, the Kauravas have forced the five Pāṇḍava brothers into exile for thirteen years despite them having the right to the throne. Actually, "forced" isn't quite right since the eldest brother lost a dice game (which may or may not have involved some trickery) and, as a result, promised to give up his kingdom. The "Preparations" section considers when it's appropriate to engage in violence. Since the Kauravas are not willing to let them return to their kingdom, the Pāṇḍavas decide to fight, but not until after a lot of negotiation and introspection. Earlier, Yudhiṣṭhira, the oldest Pāṇḍava brother, had rejected his wife Draupadī's pleas that he fight, arguing that he should keep his end of the bargain despite the sketchy circumstances of the dice game.

This lesson's sentence is the advice of the Kaurava councilor Vidura, who is advising the Kaurava king, Dhṛtarāṣṭra. It was the king's son, Prince Duryodhana, who arranged the dodgy dice game. Vidura doesn't think highly of King Dhṛtarāṣṭra in comparison to the Pāṇḍava Yudhiṣṭhira, and he says so, in a very long lecture about what makes a good king. Vidura argues that his advice isn't just pie in the sky, nice to listen to but impractical for actual ruling. He says it's both useful and follows *dharma*. To learn more about the *Mahābhārata*, see Matilal (1989) and Fitzgerald (2004).

Lesson 10

Reading: Abhidharmakośabhāṣya 9

कथं पुनरिदं गम्यते स्कन्धसन्तान एवेदमात्माभिधानं वर्तते नान्यस्मिन्नभिधेये इति । प्रत्यक्षानुमानाभावात् । . . . यदि चात्मा भवेत्तथागता एव सुव्यक्तं पशयेयुः ।

kathaṃ punar idaṃ gamyate skandhasantāna evedam ātmābhidhānaṃ vartate nānyasminn abhidheye iti. pratyakṣānumānābhāvāt . . . yadi cātmā bhavet tathāgatā eva suvyaktaṃ paśayeyuḥ.

Points of Interest For

The Curious: To learn new forms, focus mostly on the tables in 10.2.4, 6, and 7.

The Yoga Aficionado: This is our first Buddhist reading and gives arguments against the existence of the self discussed earlier; see 10.4.

The Scholar: The passive construction is very common in Sanskrit; pay attention to 10.2.5.

10.1 Vocabulary

Devanāgarī	Transliteration	Part of Speech	Translation
अन्यस्मिन्	anyasmin	masc. loc. sg. adj.	in another, in something else
अभाव	abhāva	masc. n.	absence, lack, (lit., nonbeing)
अभिधर्म	abhidharma	masc. n.	Buddhist teachings about metaphysics
अभिधान	abhidhāna	neut. n.	designation, term, word
अभिधेय	abhidheya	gerundive (future ps. ptp.)	referent, object of a word (lit., what is to be designated)
आत्मन्	ātman	masc. n.	self
कोश	kośa	masc. n.	treasury, storehouse
कथम्	katham	inter.	how (question)
√गम्	√gam	v. (1P)	understands
तथागत	tathāgata	masc. n.	the one who has gone/ come in such a way
√पश्	√paś	v. (4P)	sees, views
पुनर्	punar	indc.	then (with कथम्)
यदि	yadi	indc.	if
√वृत्	√vṛt	v. (1A)	applies to (with locative case), in the sense of a word being used for
सुव्यक्तं	suvyaktaṃ	adv.	clearly, distinctly
स्कन्ध	skandha	masc. n.	heap, aggregate

10.2 Grammar Notes

> **KEY POINT:** Verbs have moods as well as tenses. A mood tells us how to interpret a verb—as a statement of fact, a way things could be, or a command.

There's been a lot of talk about the self in this book. We've seen that early Sanskrit texts like the *Upaniṣads* suggest that there is a self that all human beings have, one which should be identified with Brahman, somehow—and this view of the self is crucial for people to come to understand. But not all Sanskrit texts agree. In fact, some think that, to adapt the words of Taylor Swift, it's *me*, the *I*, that's the problem. Buddhist philosophers like Vasubandhu, living in the fourth to fifth century CE, argue that there is no single thing that we should call "the self" (or its Sanskrit equivalent, *ātman*), and we certainly aren't identifiable with some eternally existent thing known as Brahman. In this lesson, we'll look at some reasons why they deny this self and, along the way learn two new ways to use verbs: the passive construction and the optative mood.

10.2.1 Interrogatives

> **KEY POINT:** Sanskrit interrogatives start with क् (*k*) and are (usually) case-declined to match the semantic role of the thing you're asking about.

The first word in our reading is an *interrogative*. It's a question word. "Who," "what," "when," "where," "why," and "how"—these are some of the main English interrogatives. In Sanskrit, instead of starting mostly with *w*, interrogatives start with क् (*k*). This is their basic form; as you might expect by now, they are declined, or at least many of them are. The one in our lesson, कथम् (*katham*), is not and is very common, simply meaning, "how"?

But if I want to ask *who* did something in Sanskrit, my question includes some information I expect about the answer. I ask *who*-singular (-dual, -plural) and *who*-masculine (-neuter, -feminine). For example, I might ask:

Example

Who goes?

को गच्छति ।

ko gacchati.

Notice that this form is कः (*kaḥ*) with sandhi applied. It's the same as the *a*-stem masculine declension we learned earlier in Lesson 3. I'm asking who (masculine-singular) goes. Also, notice that there is no punctuation equivalent to a question mark. Some modern editors might use them, but they're really unnecessary since the question is marked by the word कः (*kaḥ*).

Suppose I'm not sure if the sound I'm hearing, the thing I think is going, is a *who*. Maybe it's a *what*. I'd ask the same question using the neuter declension, which is somewhat unusual. It's किम् (*kim*):

Example

किं गच्छति ।

kim gacchati.

What goes?

And, finally, if I'm certain the goer takes a feminine gender, not masculine, I might ask:

Example

का गच्छति ।

kā gacchati.

Who goes?

All these forms are in the *nominative* because they're asking about the agent. However, depending on what we're asking, we would decline the interrogative differently. Just as in Lesson 3 when we built up a sentence for every role in the sentence (agent, object, etc.), we can do the same thing here. We can ask:

Example

रामः केन गच्छति ।

rāmaḥ kena gacchati.

By what does Rāma go?

Example

रामः कान् गच्छति ।

rāmaḥ kān gacchati.

To what does Rāma go?

Example

रामः कस्माद्गच्छति ।

rāmaḥ kasmād gacchati.

From what does Rāma go?

Don't forget that word order is fairly free, so you might see the interrogative at the beginning of the sentence or in other places, too. The declensions for the three genders of क (*ka*) are exactly the same as the masculine and neuter *a*-stems and feminine *ā*-stems you've learned earlier. However, for this lesson, you only need to understand कथम् (*katham*).

10.2.2 Vowel Sandhi: Final ए (e), ओ (o)

KEY POINT: Look out for "disappearing" strengthened vowels before diphthongs or non-*a* vowels.

You may have hoped we were finished with sandhi, but there are two more rules to appreciate for this lesson. The first is another disappearing vowel. Two of our strengthened vowels, ए (*e*) and ओ (*o*), change into अ (*a*) at the end of a word when they encounter any vowel or diphthong other than अ (*a*). Before अ (*a*), they stay in place, but the subsequent अ (*a*) changes into the Sanskrit "apostrophe" we learned about in Lesson 5.

Table 43. Final vowel sandhi: ए (*e*), ओ (*o*)

Final	Initial	New Final	New Initial
ए (*e*)	आ इ ई उ ऊ ओ औ ए ऐ ऋ	अ (*a*)	आ इ ई उ ऊ ओ औ ए ऐ ऋ
ओ (*o*)	आ इ ई उ ऊ ओ औ ए ऐ ऋ	अ (*a*)	आ इ ई उ ऊ ओ औ ए ऐ ऋ
ए (*e*)	अ (*a*)	ए (*e*)	ऽ (')
ओ (*o*)	अ (*a*)	ओ (*o*)	ऽ (')

Examples

कन्ये उपकुरुतः → कन्य उपकुरुतः

kanye upakurutaḥ. → kanya upakurutaḥ.

The two young women assist.

कन्ये अवगच्छतः → कन्ये ऽवगच्छतः

kanye avagacchataḥ. → kanye 'vagacchataḥ.

The two young women understand.

The possibility of "disappearing" vowels is another reason to keep an eye out for which case-ending makes sense in context.

10.2.3 Consonant Sandhi: Word-Final Doubling न् (*n*)

KEY POINT: A single final -न् (-*n*) becomes a double final -न्न् (-*nn*) when the nasal follows a short vowel and comes before a vowel starting a new word.

Our lesson illustrates another kind of sandhi: it occurs with the nasal न् (*n*) and only at the end of words. Usually the locative form of the word "other," whose stem form is अन्य (*anya*), would be अन्यस्मिन् (*anyasmin*), with only a single final -न् (*n*). But because of two conditions, it doubles: it is preceded by a short vowel, and the next sound is an initial vowel (see Table 44).

Table 44. Consonant sandhi, double final nasal

Preceding Vowel	Final Nasal	Initial Sound		Final Nasal	Example
Short vowels अ (*a*), इ (*i*), उ (*u*)	Dental nasal न् (*n*)	Any vowel	→	Doubled nasal न्न् (*nn*)	*anyasmin* + *abhidheye* → *anyasminn* + *abhidheye* अन्यस्मिन् अभिधेये → अन्यस्मिन्नभिधेये (अन्यस्मिन्न् अभिधेये)

This kind of sandhi is important to watch out for because of the similarity between a doubled -न्न् (*n*) and a single final -न् (*n*) before an initial negation, न (*na*). Sometimes, it is only by recognizing vocabulary and syntax that you can disambiguate sandhi correctly. In this example, depending on how we split sandhi, we might read the sentence in two ways:

> अन्यस्मिन्न् अभिधेये
> *anyasminn abhidheye*
> अन्यस्मिन् न भिधेये
> *anyasmin na bhidheye.*

The verb √भिद् (*bhid*) means "to cut" or, more abstractly, "to categorize," making it tempting to read this clause as involving *not dividing*.

However, the form भिधेये (*bhidheye*) isn't a grammatical way to form anything with that verb. Thus, we must conclude that sandhi is present.

10.2.4 Verbs: Ātmanepada

KEY POINT: Verbs marked with "A" are conjugated in a different pattern than those marked with "P," and sometimes the same verb can be conjugated both ways, although this doesn't always correspond to a difference in meaning.

As a gentle overview of Sanskrit, this book has only dipped into the complexities of Sanskrit verbs. Still, there's one more major idea that's worth understanding in more detail, which we introduced back in Lesson 3: the आत्मनेपद (*ātmanepada*). Verbs marked with "A" instead of "P" in the dictionary are conjugated in the *ātmanepada*, literally, "word for oneself," which is equivalent to a *middle voice*, in contrast to the *active voice* of the परस्मैपद (*parasmaipada*) ("word for another"). While there are sometimes differences in meaning between verbs in the two voices, many verbs conjugate in both voices. Today—with the exception of the passive construction (which we'll discuss below)—these are mostly different conjugation patterns and do not consistently signal differences in whether a verb is transitive or intransitive (which we discussed in Lesson 5). Below is the conjugation pattern for the thematic verbs in the present indicative:

Table 45. Present indicative verb endings, 1A

	Singular (one)	Dual (two)	Plural (more than two)
Third person (he/she/they)	-ते (-te)	-आते (-āte)	-अन्ते (-ante)
Second person (you)	-से (-se)	-आथे (-āthe)	-ध्वे (-dhve)
First person (I)	-ए (-e)	-वहे (-vahe)	-महे (-mahe)

These endings are added to our verb stem, *bhava*, which results in the pattern below (as with 1P, I omit details of sandhi and vowel lengthening, for which see any Sanskrit grammar):

Table 46. Present indicative √भू (*bhū*) (1A) - to be, to exist

	Singular	Dual	Plural
Third person	भवते (bhava**te**) - he/she/it is	भवेते (bhav**ete**) - those two are	भवन्ते (bhav**ante**) - they are
Second person	भवसे (bhava**se**) - you are	भवेथे (bhav**ethe**) - you two are	भवध्वे (bhava**dhve**) - you all are
First person	भवे (bhav**e**) - I am	भवावहे (bhavā**vahe**) - we two are	भवामहे (bhavā**mahe**) - we are

Other 1A verbs follow the same pattern, and the rest of the thematic verbs will conjugate similarly.

10.2.5 Verbs: Passive Construction

> **KEY POINT:** Sanskrit passive constructions require a passive verb with an *ātmanepada* ("A") ending and the verb's object as the grammatical subject (in the nominative).

In Lesson 9, we talked about the passive voice and the zombie test. Or, to illustrate the idea again: *the passive voice was talked about by me.* The passive voice expresses an action differently than the active voice. As we learned in Lesson 3, verbs express actions, and nouns declined in different cases express how entities are related to the action, like being the action's agent or object. In the active voice, the grammatical subject (the subject of the sentence), which is declined in the nominative, is also active:

Pattern

agent (nominative) object (accusative) verb (active)

Example

सीता राममुपकरोति ।

sītā rāmam upakaroti.

Sītā helps Rāma.

In a way, the focus here is on Sītā—she is the one acting. But in the passive voice, the focus is on the object of the action. And the object takes the nominative case—it is the *grammatical subject*, while the agent can either be entirely omitted or put in the instrumental. In the passive voice, the grammatical subject is being acted on.

Pattern

object (nominative) agent (instrumental) verb (passive)

Example

*रामः उपक्रियते ।

rāmaḥ upakriyate.[1]

Rāma is helped.

*रामः सीताया उपक्रियते ।

rāmaḥ sītāyā upakriyate.

Rāma is helped by Sīta.

1. Pandit point: I've left out the sandhi to emphasize the nominative case. But by now, you know enough to figure out what would happen to the *visarga* before this vowel. If you can't remember, go back to Lesson 5.

Even though “Rāma” is the grammatical subject—the word is in the nominative—it is passive, receiving the action. To put a verb in the passive form in Sanskrit involves the *ātmanepada* endings we’ve just learned:

Pattern

verb root + य + *ātmanepada* ending

Examples

3 sg. present passive of √कृ (*kr*) = क्रीयते (*krīyate*)

2 sg. present passive of √गम् (*gam*) = गम्यसे (*gamyase*)

Some verb roots will have phonetic changes in the root, like √कृ (*kṛ*) to क्री (*krī*), and you can find these in Whitney’s *Roots, Verb-Forms, and Primary Derivatives* or listed in many dictionaries.

10.2.6 Verbs: Optative Mood

KEY POINT: The optative mood expresses that something could or might happen and is conjugated differently than the indicative mood we’ve learned.

We have discussed verb tenses and voices so far in this book. A *tense* tells us when an action happens: Is it in the past, present, or future? A *voice* tells us about the grammatical subject of an action: Is it active or passive? Verbs also have moods. A *mood* tells us the *modality* of an action: Is it a fact, a possibility, or a command? Until now, our verbs have been *indicative*—they indicate, or state, how things are. But we can also use verbs to tell people how things might be:

Present indicative: Sītā helps Rāma.

Optative: Sītā could help Rāma.

The *optative* can be conjugated in either the *ātmanepada* or *parasmaipada* voice. Our lesson includes two examples in *parasmaipada*.

Table 47. Present optative √भू (*bhū*) (1P) - to be, to exist

	Singular	Dual	Plural
Third person	भवेत् (bhav**et**) - he/she/could be	भवेताम् (bhav**etām**) - those two could be	भवेयुः (bhav**eyuḥ**) – they could be
Second person	भवेः (bhav**eḥ**) - you could be	भवेतम् (bhav**etam**) - you two could be	भवेत (bhav**eta**) – you all could be
First person	भवेयम् (bhav**eyam**) - I could be	भवेव (bhav**eva**) – we two could be	भवेम (bhav**ema**) – we all could be

10.2.7 *an*-Stem Declension: आत्मन् (*ātman*), कर्मन् (*karman*)

This lesson is an opportunity to learn yet one more pair of useful declensions: those for nouns and adjectives ending in *-an*. We've seen examples of these words in Lesson 4 and Lesson 6, but I haven't given you the full tables. One thing to notice about the masculine version of this declension is that the stem has a strong form with a long आ (*ā*) at the end and a weak form with a final short अ (*a*). The strong forms are shaded slightly and identical forms are grouped in dark-outlined boxes.

Table 48. *an*-stem masculine, all forms (आत्मन्/*ātman*)

	Singular	Dual	Plural
Nominative	आत्मा	आत्मानौ	आत्मानः
Accusative	आत्मानम्	आत्मानौ	आत्मनः
Instrumental	आत्मना	आत्मभ्याम्	आत्मभिः
Dative	आत्मने	आत्मभ्याम्	आत्मभ्यः
Ablative	आत्मनः	आत्मभ्याम्	आत्मभ्यः
Genitive	आत्मनः	आत्मनोः	आत्मनाम्
Locative	आत्मनि	आत्मनोः	आत्मसु
Vocative	आत्मन्	आत्मानौ	आत्मानः

It's a declension very similar to कर्मन् (*karman*) and ब्रह्मन् (*brahman*), which are neuter nouns. As we've come to expect from the *a*-stem declensions, the neuter version shares the same pattern in the instrumental through locative, and the nominative, accusative, and vocative are identical. And, of course, we know enough about sandhi by now to expect changes in the nasal न् (*n*) after the र् (*r*). See Lesson 5 for a refresher.

Table 49. *an*-stem neuter, all forms (कर्मन्/*karman*)

	Singular	Dual	Plural
Nominative	कर्म	कर्मणी	कर्माणि
Accusative	कर्म	कर्मणी	कर्माणि
Instrumental	कर्मणा	कर्मभ्याम्	कर्मभिः
Dative	कर्मणे	कर्मभ्याम्	कर्मभ्यः
Ablative	कर्मणः	कर्मभ्याम्	कर्मभ्यः
Genitive	कर्मणः	कर्मणोः	कर्मणाम्
Locative	कर्मणि:	कर्मणोः	कर्मसु
Vocative	कर्म / कर्मन्	कर्मणी	कर्माणि

10.2.8 Syntax: "Carrying Over" Verbs

This next grammatical feature occurs in English and in Sanskrit, too. When two (or more) different predicates or clauses share a single verb, you can "carry over" the verb:

Example

रामो ग्रामं गच्छति न तु सीता ।

rāmo grāmaṃ gacchati na tu sītā.

Rāma goes to the town but not Sītā.

= Rāma goes to the town but Sītā [does not go to the town].

Such verb-sharing is very common in Sanskrit, and verbs can be shared a very long way across intervening words because of how cases work. Cases tip us off to the presence of an implicit verb.

10.3 Putting Everything Together

कथं पुनरिदं गम्यते स्कन्धसन्तान एवेदमात्माभिधानं वर्तते
नान्यस्मिन्नभिधेये इति । प्रत्यक्षानुमानाभावात् । . . . यदि चात्मा
भवेत्तथागता एव सुव्यक्तं पशयेयुः ।

kathaṃ punar idaṃ gamyate skandhasantāna evedam
ātmābhidhānaṃ vartate nānyasminn abhidheye iti.
pratyakṣānumānābhāvāt . . . yadi cātmā bhavet tathāgatā
eva suvyaktaṃ paśayeyuḥ.

This is a longer reading than those in previous lessons. Start by reading it aloud and making sure you understand the word boundaries.

The first sentence includes two finite verbs, one of which comes before our discourse marker इति (*iti*). Since √गम् (*gam*) has the sense of "understand," we can hypothesize that what follows it, until the *iti*—including that second verb—is part of what is understood.

We also need to pay careful attention to the vowel sandhi in this passage. Here, the verb √वृत् (*vṛt*) is being used in the sense of a word's application for or about some object, and so we expect a locative case ending. This will help us confirm we've restored sandhi correctly. We can carry over the verb from the first clause to the second, which has two words with locative case endings. In this clause, though, we will negate the verb with न (*na*), which we discussed in Lesson 5. Finally, our second sentence is a single compound ending with -अभावात् (*-abhāvāt*). The ablative case here signals that Vasubandhu is giving a reason: because of the absence (अभाव/*abhāva*) of something.

The next part of the reading is a sentence from later in the chapter, in which Vasubandhu gives us another reason for what is embedded in the *iti*-clause. This reason uses the optative mood to describe how things *would be*. The implication is that things aren't this way: compare someone who says, "If a pig had wings, it could fly." They aren't saying that pigs have wings.

In this last sentence, sandhi is important for identifying the subject (gender, case, and number). But since we have a verb, this helps us, too—the subject and the verb must match in number. Finally, remember that adverbs like सुव्यक्तम् (*suvyaktam*) modify verbs.

With these hints, try to read the two clauses in the second sentence—be sure to identify the subject of each. Remember that this is supposed to give a reason for how things *would* be under certain circumstances, but aren't actually.

10.4 About the Reading: No Selves, Just *Skandhas*

Vasubandhu, the author of this lesson's text, lived centuries after the historical Buddha, whose given name was Gautama. The Buddha didn't write any Buddhist texts we have today, and certainly not in Sanskrit—the earliest are in a related language, Pali (or "Pāḷi"). But by the fourth century CE, when Vasubandhu wrote his *Abhidharmakośa* (*Treasury of Buddhist Metaphysics*) and his autocommentary (*bhāṣya*), Sanskrit was a more common choice for Buddhist thinkers. Scholars don't know precisely why Buddhists began to write in Sanskrit more often, but some, drawing on what Vasubandhu himself says, think it's because this was a language that would give them credibility with their brahmanical interlocutors.[2]

Our reading comes from the ninth chapter of the *Abhidharmakośabhāṣya*, which is Vasubandhu's own commentary on the verses, or *kārikas*, which he wrote. Interestingly, though, the ninth chapter doesn't have any verses. It's

2. This is what Eltschinger (2017) argues. He cites Vasubandhu's remark about the usefulness of studying the Sanskrit language: it allows "him who studies it to '[use] well-formed expressions and [to arouse] other peoples' confidence" (321).

a prose-only discussion of why Buddhists should reject the idea of a self or a soul—Vasubandhu is equally adamant that there is no immaterial entity like a soul and that there is no permanently enduring physical thing we call a "self." Instead, he argues that what we mistakenly call a "self" is just a series of aggregates. The word for "aggregate" is स्कन्ध (*skandha*). More colloquially, it means "heap." These heaps are just bunches of feelings, physical parts, thoughts, conscious experiences, and inclinations (or "dispositions"). Since these things all change from moment to moment, and there is no underlying single thing that remains the same throughout an entire life, there is no self.

Even though I use the word "Malcolm" to talk about my "self" from birth to death, there is no single thing that stays the same from birth to death, Vasubandhu would say: no invisible, immaterial soul and no part of my body or experience, either. The thing I'm talking about is like a filmstrip or—to update the analogy—a digital video. Each frame is composed of pixels (aggregated together). And the video is just a series of changing pixels. That's you and me. And while we can talk about the "movie" or "moving picture," no *thing* is moving. That's an illusion. There are just pixels that appear rapidly in different configurations.

The first two sentences in the lesson have an interlocutor ask why we should believe this central Buddhist idea. The second sentence comes much later in the chapter and gives an additional reason for believing there is no self. Interestingly, in this chapter, Vasubandhu is arguing with a group of Buddhists who want to accept the reality of a person but deny the existence of a self. They're trying to split the difference, accepting that there is something, a "person," which really exists, although it exists in the sense of a useful fiction. These persons aren't the same thing as the always-changing heaps. But, these "Personalist" Buddhists argue, they're also not something entirely different. Vasubandhu isn't convinced, and in our lesson, he gives several reasons why we shouldn't accept a self or a person.[3]

3. For more discussion of Vasubandhu's arguments, see Gold (2022).

Lesson 11

Reading: Rājamartaṇḍa 1.2

को योग इत्यत आह
योगश्चित्तवृत्तिनिरोधः ॥ १।२ ॥
चित्तस्यान्तःकरणस्य
वक्ष्यमाणा या वृत्तयस्तासां
निरोधो निर्वर्त्तनं योग इत्यर्थः।

ko yoga ity ata āha
yogaś cittavṛttinirodhaḥ (1.2)
cittasyāntaḥkaraṇasya vakṣyamāṇā yā
vṛttayastāsāṃ nirodho
nirvarttanaṃ yoga ity arthaḥ.

Points of Interest For

The Curious: Focus on reading about what commentaries do. Leave the reading as a challenge to come back to later if you'd like.

The Yoga Aficionado: Look out for a discussion of the *Bhagavadgītā* and an important early commentary on it in section 11.2.3.

The Scholar: Go back to the second lesson and compare how you understood *Yogasūtra* 2 with how our commentator understands it, focusing especially on the analysis of the compounds.

11.1 Vocabulary

Devanāgarī	Transliteration	Part of Speech	Translation
अक्ष	akṣa	neut. n.	sense faculty
अनुमान	anumāna	neut. n.	inference
अन्तःकरण	antaḥkaraṇa	neut. n.	internal faculty (like the mind)
अभिप्राय	abhiprāya	masc. n.	thought, idea
आक्षिपति	ākṣipati	pres. indc. 3 sg from आ + √क्षिप् (6P)	he/she/one replies, responds
आह	āha	v. perfect 3 sg. from √अह् (reconstructed form)	he/she/one says
उपमान	upamāna	neut. n.	comparison, analogy
कण्ठ	kaṇṭha	masc. n.	throat, neck
कन्या	kanyā	fem. noun	girl, young woman
कीकस	kīkasa	neut. n.	bone
चेत्	cet	indc.	could be, might be (with *iti*)
तात्पर्य	tātparya	neut. n.	intention, aim
ननु	nanu	indc.	discourse marker indicating objection in what follows: "But couldn't it be that?," "is it not that"
निर्वर्त्तन	nirvarttana	neut. n.	accomplishing, completing

पदच्छेद	padaccheda	masc. n.	word-division
पुत्र	putra	masc. n.	son
प्रज्ञा	prajñā	fem. n.	knowledge, wisdom
प्रति	prati	pfx.	toward, for; for each
प्रतिष्ठिता	pratiṣṭhitā	fem. nom. sg. ppp. (as adj. from प्रति + √स्था, 1P)	being in a fixed, firm state
प्रमाण	pramāṇa	neut. n.	way of knowing, knowledge source
भावः	bhāva	masc. n.	meaning, idea (esp. with *iti*)
मुख	mukha	neut. n.	face, mouth
वाक्ष्यमाणाः	vākṣyamāṇāḥ	future ptp., fem. nom. pl. from √वच् (2P)	what will be said later, what needs to be mentioned
विग्रह	vigraha	masc. n.	analysis (of compound), separation into its parts
विषय	viṣaya	masc. n.	object, content of an experience
शब्द	śabda	masc. n.	speech, language, testimony
शेष	śeṣa	masc. n.	remainder, what must be supplied (with *iti*)
स्थित	sthita	ppp. (as adj. from √स्था, 1P)	being in a particular state

11.2 What Commentaries Do

KEY POINT: A Sanskrit commentary explains another text by breaking sandhi for word division, giving word meanings, analyzing compounds, paraphrasing sentence meanings, and responding to potential objections and points of confusion.

Sanskrit texts can be difficult, as we've seen. And they aren't only difficult for modern Sanskrit readers. Many Sanskrit students find themselves reassured when they discover that a commentator is just as puzzled as they are by a grammatical construction or turn of phrase. Seeing that others have found some material hard may not immediately help you understand it. But, when expert readers, deeply immersed in the language and literature of Sanskrit, disagree about how to understand vocabulary or split sandhi, it's comforting. (Or perhaps it's a case of schadenfreude, that useful German word for enjoying another person's suffering.)

More often, though, Sanskrit commentators are in a position to help the modern reader. Not only are these authors experts in the language but they are also embedded in the culture and traditions that inform these texts. Sometimes, they are distant from the original text by many hundreds of years, which means they do not have a perfect understanding of the author's original intention—when the text has a single author. And sometimes, commentators disagree among themselves. But consulting a commentary enriches our experience of reading Sanskrit and can help us refine our understanding of its grammar, semantic range, and beauty.

So, what is a commentary? Most generally, a commentary explains another text. As we saw in Lesson 2, the style of writing known as सूत्र (*sūtra*) is very compressed. Commentaries expand these *sūtras*. For a long time in Sanskrit literature—whether philosophy, grammar, poetry, or law—commentary was one of the primary ways later writers discussed earlier writing. Instead of writing essays (a genre originating in the French Renaissance), authors would write commentaries on earlier work.

Sometimes, these commentaries put more effort into developing the new author's own ideas and responding to objections and replies than explaining the original text. However, commentaries almost always show deference to the original text (known as a *root text*), even if their interpretations seem awkward.[1] In these cases, commentators argued their "new" ideas were recovering some "lost" or "hidden" meaning in the original text. Although there are many different kinds of commentaries, here we will focus on understanding and illustrating five common methods.[2]

11.2.1 Word Division

> **KEY POINT:** Commentators break sandhi for readers, especially when there are multiple ways to do so that impact meaning.

From the very beginning of this book, you have learned about the importance of sandhi in reading Sanskrit. It's no coincidence that separating words at their boundaries, or पदच्छेद (*padaccheda*) is the first thing a commentary is described as doing.[3] If commentators discussed every instance of sandhi, commentaries would be a tedious slog, indeed! However, typically, they assume that we can split most sandhi. Their explicit discussions on this topic usually happen only when there is a puzzling case, such as when multiple options exist and would impact our understanding. For instance, as we saw at the end of Lesson 6, by splitting

---

1. For a survey of different kinds of commentary, see Preisendanz (2008).

2. See Tubb and Boose (2007) for a detailed discussion of these five "services."

3. Pandit point: A classic statement of these services is from the पराशरपुराण (*Parāśarapurāṇa*): "The five characteristics of an explanation are: the separation of words, the statement of word-meanings, compound-division, construing sentences, settling objections."

पदच्छेदः पदार्थोक्तिर्विग्रहो वाक्ययोजना ।
आक्षेपेषु समाधाणं व्याख्यानं पञ्चलक्षणम् ॥
padacchedaḥ padārthoktir vigraho vākyayojanā |
ākṣepeṣu samādhāṇaṃ vyākhyānaṃ pañcalakṣaṇam ||
(Quoted in Tubb and Boose [2007, 3]).

vowel sandhi (and inserting a stop or | in different places), we can get two diametrically opposed interpretations:

Root text

स आत्मातत्त्वमसि ।

sa ātmātattvamasi.

Word-division 1

स आत्मा । अतत् त्वम् असि ।

sa ātmā. atat tvam asi.

This is the self. You are not-that.

Word-division 2

स आत्मा तत् त्वम् असि ।

sa ātmā tat tvam asi.

This is the self, that which you are.

While these ambiguities aren't always so significant, authors and commentators can play on them to great literary effect, especially in poetry—as we'll see in the next lesson.

And commentaries often repeat the words in the root text, which will help you with the sandhi. For this reason, if you're reading a text, you might look at a commentary to see where to split words. We'll see examples in the next section.

11.2.2 Word Meaning

> **KEY POINT:** Glossing word meanings is a way to help readers understand vocabulary.

Sanskrit commentators constantly *gloss*, that is, present synonyms of, or explanations for, words. They do this in a similar way as I just did in English. I used the phrase "that is," along with a phrase set apart by commas, to gloss the word "gloss."

The practice of glossing is why many Sanskrit instructors suggest beginning students read with a print version of a text, pencil in hand. This helps you easily underline words in the commentary that appear in the root text.[4]

Many printed editions will bold the Sanskrit text where the editor has identified these glosses, which can be helpful, although they may not identify all of them. Here is an example from the *Nyāyabhāṣya*, the commentary that Vātsyāyana wrote on the *Nyāyasūtra*.[5] I've bolded the *sūtra* text. The commentary is below it.

Example

प्रत्यक्षानुमानोपमानशब्दाः प्रमाणानि ।

अक्षस्याक्षस्य प्रतिविषयं वृत्तिः प्रत्यक्षम् ।

pratyakṣānumānopamānaśabdāḥ pramāṇāni.

akṣasyākṣasya prativiṣayaṃ vṛttiḥ pratyakṣam.

The first thing I would do while reading the commentary is to underline the word *pratyakṣam* because the word *pratyakṣa-* appears in the *sūtra* as part of a compound. So, I suspect it's being glossed:

Example

अक्षस्याक्षस्य प्रतिविषयं वृत्तिः <u>प्रत्यक्षम्</u> ।

akṣasyākṣasya prativiṣayaṃ vṛttiḥ <u>pratyakṣam</u>.

4. Of course, there are ways to do this with technology. You can annotate PDFs or documents as you read. The idea is just to slow down and pay attention to the text. And the use of hyperlinks in digital Sanskrit texts can structure the text in ways that commentaries do. However, I think many Sanskrit instructors are suspicious that over-reliance on digital tools may prevent beginning students from internalizing key ideas since the thinking remains "outsourced" to external tools. (Sanskritists are involved in some very technical projects in the digital humanities, so to characterize the discipline as anti-technological would be a gross overgeneralization.)

5. For a translation of this section, see Dasti and Phillips (2017, 17).

Suppose, when reading the *sūtra*, I wasn't sure whether I should split the compound as *pratyakṣā-anumāna-* or *pratyakṣa-anumāna-*. Because Vātsyāyana declines the word as *pratyakṣam*, I split it the second way, as this declension follows the *a*-stem pattern for a masculine noun in the accusative or a neuter noun in the nominative or accusative and not a feminine *ā*-stem pattern (go back to Lesson 9 for a refresher—and note that the noun is, in fact, neuter). This is how the first and second functions of commentaries work together.

Vātsyāyana has glossed the word *pratyakṣa* in a way you will encounter a lot in commentaries. He has analyzed the word's component parts, *praty* + *akṣa*. (Quick check before you move on: What vowel would turn into a *y* before an *a*? Go back to Lesson 6 if you can't remember!)

The prefix *prati-* has a lot of meanings. Often it means "toward," "for," or "onto." But it can also have a *distributive* sense, as in "for every" or "for each." This latter sense is how Vātsyāyana understands the prefix, which we know through his repetition of the word अक्ष (*akṣa*) in the neuter genitive singular. (The word अक्ष (*akṣa*) means "sense"— like our eyesight or our hearing.)

This repetition is a pattern we haven't seen before. It conveys the idea of distribution. Think of the lines in "The Rime of the Ancient Mariner," "water, water, every where, / Nor any drop to drink." Here, "water" doesn't mean two bits of water—it's suggesting the vast ocean. All the water. Similarly, here we can translate the repeated "of the sense faculty, of the sense faculty" with the word "each" instead of translating both words:

Example

अक्षस्याक्षस्य प्रतिविषयं वृत्तिः ।

akṣasyākṣasya prativiṣayaṃ vṛttiḥ.

the operating (*vṛttiḥ*) upon each object (*prativiṣayaṃ*) of each sense faculty (*akṣasyākṣasya*)

And, as we learned all the way back in Lesson 2, nominal sentences are common in Sanskrit, so we can translate this as:

Example

अक्षस्याक्षस्य प्रतिविषयं वृत्तिः प्रत्यक्षम् ।

akṣasyākṣasya prativiṣayaṃ vṛttiḥ pratyakṣam.

The operating (*vṛttiḥ*) of each sense faculty (*akṣasyākṣasya*) upon each object (*prativiṣayaṃ*) is "perception" (*pratyakṣam*).

I've put the word "perception" in quotes to show Vātsyāyana is explaining the first word of the *sūtra*. We could also reorder the sentence since in English, we'd often start with the word we're glossing and add "each respective" to make clear that the single object is one for every sense faculty (eyesight functions on visible things, hearing on audible things, etc.):

Example

अक्षस्याक्षस्य प्रतिविषयं वृत्तिः प्रत्यक्षम् ।

akṣasyākṣasya prativiṣayaṃ vṛttiḥ pratyakṣam.

"Perception" is the operating of each sense faculty upon each respective object.

There is one last point, which we'll discuss further in Lesson 13. Translators will make the functions of a commentary more explicit by various strategies. Here's how Matthew Dasti and Stephen Phillips handle this sentence:

> To follow the etymology of the word, **perception** (*pratyakṣa*) is the functioning of each *sense faculty* (*akṣa*) upon its *own proper* (*praty*) object. . . .[6]

They've inserted the phrase, "to follow the etymology of the word," to help readers understand what the commentary is doing—glossing by breaking the word *pratyakṣa* into its parts. Commentators gloss words in many ways, and to learn about them, you should consult chapter 3 of

6. Dasti and Phillips (2017, 17). See Lesson 13 for a discussion of different translation strategies.

Tubb and Boose (2007). However, to get you started, below are a few key terms which come after a gloss:

> इत्यर्थः (*ity arthaḥ*) – "this is the meaning"[7]
> इति भावः (*iti bhāvaḥ*) – "this is the idea"
> इत्यभिप्रायः (*ity abhiprāyaḥ*), इति तात्पर्यः (*iti tātparyaḥ*) – "this is the intention"
> इति यावत् (*iti yāvat*) – "this is specifically the meaning"

11.2.3 Compound Analysis

KEY POINT: Compounds in the root text are analyzed in the commentary when their component parts get split apart and declined endings are restored.

The analysis of compounds in Sanskrit is called विग्रह (*vigraha*). Because there is a vast and sophisticated grammatical literature in Sanskrit, commentators can delve deeply into compounds and other forms. Sometimes, they will cite grammatical authorities such as Pāṇini, who lived around the fifth century BCE—and whose name you now know is *not* pronounced like the Italian sandwich, the panini. An introduction to Pāṇini's work is well beyond this book's scope.[8] Even though commentaries analyze a range of grammatical forms, we will look only at compounds, and of these, just two which we've focused on in this book: the determinative compound and the exocentric compound.[9]

7. Pandit point: Again, remember that Devanāgarī will print words together even when they are not compounds. So you will commonly see इत्यर्थः even though it is transliterated *ity arthaḥ*.

8. In addition to Tubb and Boose (2007, chap. 4), for more on Pāṇini, see Cardona (1988) and a searchable version of Pāṇini's work, the *Aṣṭādhyāyī* (*Eight Chapters*), hosted by Sanskritdictionary.com, https://sanskritdictionary.com/panini/.

9. There are many kinds of compounds and lots of ways to gloss them in commentaries. Again, see Tubb and Boose (2007, esp. chaps. 8, 13) for more.

Compounds

Analyzing compounds, at its simplest, is just separating the component parts and adding the case endings that have been omitted:

Pattern

Compound: $word_1word_2$*+ending*

Analysis: ($word_1$*+ending*) + ($word_2$*+ending*)

Example

Compound: देवपुत्रः (*devaputraḥ*)

Analysis: देवस्य पुत्रः (*devasya putraḥ*)

The example shows that the masculine genitive singular ending -स्य (*-sya*) has been restored. This means the son is of a single god, not many gods. If the compound were interpreted as "the son of the *gods*," it would be analyzed:

Example

Compound: देवपुत्रः (*devaputraḥ*)

Analysis: देवानां पुत्रः (*devānāṃ putraḥ*)

We also know that the compound is a *dependent determinative compound*. In other words, it means "the son *of* the god" and not "the son *that is* a god," a *descriptive determinative compound*. If the compound were "the son that is a god," it would be analyzed differently:

Example

Compound: देवपुत्रः (*devaputraḥ*)

Analysis: देवः पुत्रः (*devaḥ putraḥ*)

Here, the gender, case, and number are the same: masculine, nominative, and singular. Sometimes, commentators will identify multiple candidates for interpreting the compound. And commentators may disagree with each other, too.

Another kind of compound you'll see analyzed is the *exocentric compound*. To appreciate this form of analysis, you might want to refresh your memory about relative and correlative forms found in Lesson 8. That's because these are an essential part of this *vigraha*.

Pattern

Compound: $word_1word_2$

Analysis: One who has a $word_1$-ending $word_2$-ending is a "$word_1word_2$."

English Example

Compound: redcoat

Analysis: One whose coat is red is a "redcoat."

The analysis shows us that "redcoat" is not referring to a coat that is red but to the person who owns the red coat.

Sanskrit Example (simple)

Compound: नीलकण्ठः (*nīlakaṇṭhaḥ*)

Analysis: नीलः कण्ठो यस्य स नीलकण्ठः ।

nīlaḥ kaṇṭho yasya sa nīlakaṇṭhaḥ.

The one (*saḥ*) who has (*yasya*) a throat that is black (*nīlaḥ kaṇṭhaḥ*) is "a black-throat."

Like the case of "redcoat," the analysis makes it clear that "black-throat" is not referring to a throat that is black, but someone, like the god Śiva, who has a black throat. The compound itself might be analyzed differently, too. This example is of a *descriptive* determinative compound, but we also can perform a similar analysis for *dependent* determinative compounds like this one:

Sanskrit Example (simple)

Compound: वीरसेनः (*vīrasenaḥ*)

Analysis: vīrāṇāṃ senā यस्य स वीरसेनः ।

vīrāṇāṃ senā yasya sa vīrasenaḥ.

The one (*saḥ*) who has (*yasya*) an army (*senā*) that is made of heroes (*vīrāṇām*) is "Hero Army."[10]

Once we appreciate the basic structure of a compound analysis, we can understand more complex ones, which include etymological glosses. Here is an example from Śaṅkara's commentary on the *Bhagavadgītā*:

Sanskrit Example (complex)

Compound: स्थितप्रज्ञस्य (*sthitaprajñasya*, masc. gen. sg.)

Analysis: ***स्थिता** प्रतिष्ठिता अहम् अस्मि परं ब्रह्म इति प्रज्ञा यस्य सः **स्थितप्रज्ञः**।

***sthitā** pratiṣṭhitā aham asmi paraṃ brahma iti prajñā yasya saḥ **sthitaprajñaḥ**.[11]

The one for whom (*yasya*) the knowledge (*prajña*) "I am the supreme Brahman," is "fixed" (*sthitā*), that is, *firmly* fixed (*pratiṣṭhitā*), that one (*saḥ*) is the "one whose knowledge is fixed."

In this more complex example, Śaṅkara explains a compound in the *Bhagavadgītā* 2.54. He combines glossing with compound analysis, glossing the term स्थित- (*sthita*) in the compound with प्रतिष्ठिता (*pratiṣṭhitā*).

---

10. Pandit point: This is an epithet for a character in the Mahābhārata, as well as some living people. There are also a lot of compound names for birds and other animals. A bird is "nest-born" (नीडज, *nīḍa-ja*), "a cloud-goer" (अभ्रग, *abhra-ga*), "one whose house is in a tree" (वृक्षगृह, *vṛkṣa-gṛha*). An elephant is "a circle-foot" (चक्रपाद, *cakra-pāda*), and a lion is "the lord of the animals" (गणेश्वर, *gaṇeśvara*). English doesn't have as many of these, except for specific kinds of animals, like birds: yellowthroats are birds whose throats are yellow. Internet culture has begun to create some compound names for animals, like "danger noodle" for snakes, though this is not a *bahuvrīhi*, as discussed in Lesson 5. (Challenge: How would you analyze "danger noodle," based on the compound categories you've learned?) It adds another layer of complexity since it's metaphorical (snakes look like noodles). We'll see comparison and compounds together in Lesson 12.

11. Here's the example with complete sandhi: स्थिता प्रतिष्ठिता अहमस्मि परं ब्रह्म इति प्रज्ञा यस्य सः स्थितप्रज्ञः।
*sthitā pratiṣṭhitā ahamasmi paraṃ brahma iti prajñā yasya saḥ sthitaprajñaḥ.

Because the word for knowledge is feminine, so too are the adjectives for the kind of knowledge (स्थिता/*sthitā*, प्रतिष्ठिता/*pratiṣṭhitā*). This is despite the fact that in the verse, the word is an exocentric compound, referring to *someone* who has this kind of knowledge (and that person is a man or at least referred to with a generic masculine gender). Śaṅkara also explains what the knowledge is—for him, there is a particular thing which the स्थितप्रज्ञ (*sthitaprajña*) must know about Brahman. Notice how we are able to tell that the first two words aren't part of the *iti*-clause (what is being quoted): not only is it customary to start glossing with the first word, but also there is no grammatical relationship between the complete sentence (*अहम् अस्मि परं ब्रह्म, *aham asmi paraṃ brahma*) and the two feminine gender nouns, (स्थिता प्रतिष्ठिता, *sthitā pratiṣṭhitā*).

11.2.4 Sentence Meaning

KEY POINTS: Commentators explain the structure of sentences and larger sections of the text by inserting material; they also paraphrase sentences and explain their meanings.

The list of *iti*-s at the end of 11.2.2 can also signal when a commentator is explaining the meaning of a sentence. And commentaries don't just explain the meanings of sentences; they also explain their order. Here's an analogy: accomplished bakers easily understand a terse recipe because they are familiar with other recipes and are competent with usual ingredients, their ratios, and baking techniques:

> Heat oven to 350 F
>
> Whip butter, sugar
>
> Add vanilla and egg, flour, baking soda, salt, and chocolate chips
>
> Scoop onto trays
>
> Bake until done

But the connections between steps are implicit, as are the full meanings of each step. What kind of oven should we use? How much of each ingredient? What's the best way to measure? How big are the scoops? How do we know when a cookie is done? A fuller explanation might be:

> Heat oven to 350. Why begin with this step? The purpose is to preheat the oven to 350 F, where "F" means "Fahrenheit," while preparing the ingredients to allow the oven time to reach temperature. You might wonder, what is the first thing to do after turning on the oven? This is why the recipe says next, "Whip butter, sugar." What "whip butter, sugar" really means is that you should make *softened* butter *and then add* sugar *to* the butter.

This illustrates two techniques commentaries use to unpack structure: inserting questions between *sūtras*, like "Why begin with this step?" and inserting words and phrases within sentences, like "softened" and "and then add."

Inserting questions between sentences

We learned about questions in Lesson 10. The imaginary example above illustrates how commentaries use rhetorical questions. These questions may be ones that philosophical opponents would raise, or they may simply be clarifying questions, like a student would ask.

Inserting words into sentences

Commentators will insert material that they think needs to be supplied in the original text, and they will insert little additional phrases to clarify what's going on. One useful phrase to know, to add to your stock of *iti*-s is:

> **Pattern**
> इति शेषः (*iti śeṣaḥ*)
>
> "this is supplied"

Sanskrit Example

रामो ग्रामं गच्छति । *अश्वेन इति शेषः ।

rāmo grāmaṃ gacchati. *aśvena iti śeṣaḥ.[12]

Rāma goes to the town. Supply "by horse."

11.2.5 Objections and Replies

> **KEY POINT:** Commentators consider actual or possible objections to the text and then respond to them.

Especially for philosophical Sanskrit texts, raising objections and replies is a central part of the commentary. Of course, unless we know what the *sūtra* text says, we can't respond to objections. This makes the first four commentarial functions important. But many commentators will spend pages upon pages raising and responding to objections and relatively less time on the grammar of the root text. Yet another *iti* helps us recognize when this is happening:

Pattern

sentence इति चेत् (*iti cet*). न (*na*).

One might think, "sentence." No.

Or:

One might think that sentence. No.

Example

रामः रथेन ग्रामं गच्छतीति चेत् । न ।

rāmaḥ rathena grāmaṃ gacchatīti cet. na.

One might think that Rāma goes to the town by chariot. No.

12. Pandit point: With sandhi: अश्वेनेति शेषः (*aśveneti śeṣaḥ*).

Another common word that identifies an objection is ननु (*nanu*).[13] Often translators will just use the word "objection" or "objector" to mark this phrase, though it can also be translated as a question, "But couldn't it be . . . ?"

Pattern

ननु (*nanu*) sentence

But couldn't it be, "sentence"?

[Objection:] "sentence."

Example

ननु रामः प्लवेन ग्रामं गच्छतीति चेत् । न ।

nanu rāmaḥ plavena grāmaṃ gacchatīti cet. na.

But couldn't it be that one might think Rāma goes to the town by boat? No.

The previous function often combines with this one. Commentators might insert these markers to show us that one *sūtra* raises an objection and another replies to it. You will encounter many synonyms for "object" and "reply" that use इति (*iti*). Our last example illustrates Śaṅkara's introduction to the first verse in Lesson 13, *Bhagavadgītā* 3.14.

Pattern

sentence. इत्युच्यते (*ity ucyate*)

sentence. To this, it is said . . .[14]

---

13. Pandit point: Sometimes Sanskrit authors quote objections verbatim; other times, they paraphrase or allude to different texts. But we can't always identify a particular objector or textual origin. It seems that Sanskrit philosophers consider possible responses just like modern philosophers.

14. Pandit point: This form is the passive construction in the third person for the verb √वच् (*vac*), 2P. It has a weak stem to which the passive marker य (*-ya*) is added. While literally you might translate, "it is said," English uses the passive less frequently, so translators often opt for an active version, like "we say" or "one says."

Example

जगच्चक्रप्रवृत्तिहेतुर्हि कर्म । कथम् । इत्युच्यते ।

jagaccakrapravṛttihetur hi karma. katham. ity ucyate.

For activity is the cause (*hetu*) of turning (*pravṛtti*) the universe's wheel (*jagat-cakra*). How? To this, it is said:

You can see these small words do a lot of work in commentaries.

11.3 Putting Everything Together

को योग इत्यत आह

योगश्चित्तवृत्तिनिरोधः ॥ १।२ ॥

चित्तस्यान्तःकरणस्य वक्ष्यमाणा या वृत्तयस्तासां निरोधो निर्वर्त्तनं योग इत्यर्थः।

ko yoga ity ata āha

yogaś cittavṛttinirodhaḥ (1.2)

cittasyāntaḥkaraṇasya vakṣyamāṇā yā vṛttayastāsāṃ nirodho nirvarttanaṃ **yoga** ity arthaḥ.

This reading is from the tenth-century commentator Bhoja Rāja, whose work is less well-known but grammatically simpler than the more famous *Yogabhāṣya* (*Commentary on Yoga*) attributed to Vyāsa. The *Rājamartaṇḍa* (*The Royal Sun*) is, strictly speaking, a commentary on Vyāsa's text. This makes it a *sub*-commentary. We can have many layers of commentaries on commentaries on commentaries. (And some authors write "commentaries" on their own verses, which are *auto*-commentaries.) Our example focuses on a portion of the *Rājamartaṇḍa* that comments directly on the *sūtra* we saw in Lesson 2, not on Vyāsa's commentary.

In this commentary, we see Bhoja introducing the *sūtra* and explaining a crucial term. (I have bolded the term and the verse.) He begins with a question, "What is yoga?" The end of his question is marked with our familiar discourse particle इति (*iti*). By supplying this question, Bhoja interprets the point of the second verse of the *Yogasūtra*: it's to answer someone who wonders this. Bhoja makes this interpretation explicit with the indeclinable अतः (*ataḥ*), whose *visarga* has dropped due to sandhi. Having introduced the *sūtra*, Bhoja reproduces it—now you should be able to read this verse easily! But what does it mean?

Bhoja helps us out with a sentence that gives us the meaning. We know this because it ends with इत्यर्थः (*ity arthaḥ*). His gloss restates the definition by explaining the parts of the compound in the order in which they appear: चित्तवृत्तिनिरोधः (*citta-vṛtti-nirodhaḥ*). For each component word, he gives us the case ending and then its meaning.

He understands चित्त (*citta-*) to be चित्तस्य (*cittasya*), "of the mind." And another word for चित्तस्य (*cittasya*) is अन्तःकरणस्य (*antaḥkaraṇasya*). As a genitive, what does चित्तस्य (*cittasya*) belong to? The वृत्ति (*vṛtti-*), which is the next word in the compound.

And there is not just one वृत्तिः (*vṛttiḥ*), but many: वृत्तयः (*vṛttayaḥ*)—remember our *visarga* sandhi with sibilants and dentals, from Lesson 2. This feminine nominative plural term isn't given a synonym, but Bhoja promises it is something that will be talked about: the text reads वक्ष्यमाणाः याः (*vakṣyamāṇāḥ yāḥ*) with our sandhi restored.

What about the head of the compound, निरोधः (*-nirodhaḥ*)? Bhoja explains that it is of these तासाम् (*tāsām*) that there is cessation. "These" refers back to the activities. There is the cessation, singular (*nirodaḥ*) of these activities. The word निर्वर्त्तनम् *nirvarttanam* derives from निर् (*nir*) and √वृत् (*vṛt*), which makes the connection to the many वृत्तयः (*vṛttayaḥ*) clear. It's like saying, "yoga de-*activates* mental *activities*." Below is a word-by-word analysis of the passage. Putting this together into intelligible English is your challenge. Go back through the commentary and verse from start to finish, breaking sandhi and reading units of the reading one at a time—reference Table 50 to help you with this passage.

Table 50. Analysis of *Rājamartaṇḍa*

Sanskrit (Sandhi Restored)	Gloss (Grammatical Analysis)
cittasya	of the mind (neut. gen. sg.)
antaḥkaraṇasya	of the internal faculty (neut. gen. sg.)
vakṣyamāṇāḥ yāḥ vṛttayaḥ	that which will be discussed (fem. nom. pl.) the activities (fem. nom. pl)
tāsāṃ	of these (fem. gen. pl.)
nirodhaḥ	cessation (masc. nom. sg.)
nirvarttanam	activity-ending (neut. nom. sg.)
yogaḥ	yoga (masc. nom. sg.)

Keep in mind that there are nominal sentences in Sanskrit and that Bhoja is trying to explain the *sūtra*. You might need to insert helping verbs and use quotation marks.

11.4 About the Reading: Deactivating Mental Activities

Bhoja's commentary explains that the practice of *yoga* aims to stop mental activities. Human beings need this "deactivation" because they have mistaken their true self—which is pure consciousness—with *un*conscious processes like thought and emotion. There is not only one mental activity, or a few, like negative thoughts or unhealthy attachments, that we are supposed to stop, according to the *Yogasūtra*. Mental activities, in general, should stop. Bhoja's unpacking of the compound makes this clear—it is activities, plural, that should cease.

This idea that mental activities are not conscious is unusual for modern people, who typically identify consciousness with the mental. But, as we saw in Lesson 2, Bhoja and other commentators divide the world into conscious and unconscious differently: pure consciousness does not change, like mental processes do, constantly. Bryant (2015) says much more about this topic, along with discussion of the classical commentators.

11.5 Further Resources

Probably the most accessible online introduction to reading Sanskrit commentaries is Guy Leavitt's website, designed for his Columbia University Sanskrit courses. There, he has an example of commentary on Sanskrit poetry or काव्य (*kāvya*) written by Jonarāja, a fifteenth-century CE Kashmiri literary theorist who writes on the श्रीकण्ठचरित (*Śrīkaṇṭhacarita*), a highly philosophical poem by Maṅkhaka in the twelfth century CE. (Lesson 12 includes some discussion of Sanskrit poetry.)

> Leavitt, Guy. "Commentary." Introductory Sanskrit. Accessed October 2, 2022. http://www.introductory-sanskrit.com/commentary.html.

For a comprehensive reference guide, Tubb and Boose's *Scholastic Sanskrit* is a matchless resource. The introductory material for each section details how commentaries function, and the book includes examples from a range of Sanskrit commentaries. (Note that their transliteration style uses different conventions from this book—see Lesson 13 for details.)

> Tubb, Gary Alan, and Emery Robert Boose. *Scholastic Sanskrit: A Handbook for Students*. New York: American Institute of Buddhist Studies, 2007.

Overlapping some with the above resources—but going beyond them in explaining the different types of commentaries and some history of their conception in Sanskrit literature—is Jonardon Ganeri's paper, which, as of this writing, is hosted online by Columbia University.

> Ganeri, Jonardon. "Sanskrit Philosophical Commentary." *Journal of the Indian Council of Philosophical Research* 27 (2010): 187–207. Online preprint version hosted at http://ftp.columbia.edu/itc/mealac/pollock/sks/papers/Ganeri(commentary).pdf.

Lesson 12

Reading: Raghuvaṃśa 1.1

वागर्थाविव संपृक्तौ वागर्थप्रतिपत्तये ।
जगतः पितरौ वन्दे पार्वतीपरमेश्वरौ ॥ १।१

वागर्थाविव शब्दार्थाविव संपृक्तौ नित्यसंबद्धावित्यर्थः । जगतो लोकस्य पितरौ। माता च पिता च पितरौ । पार्वती च परमेश्वरशश्च पार्वतीपरमेश्वरौ ।

vāgarthāv iva sampṛktau vāgarthapratipattaye |
jagataḥ pitarau vande
pārvatīparameśvarau || 1.1
vāgarthāv iva śabdārthāv iva saṃpṛktau nityasaṃbaddhāv ity arthaḥ. jagato lokasya pitarau. mātā ca pitā ca pitarau. pārvatī ca parameśvaraśaś ca pārvatīparameśvarau.

Points of Interest For

The Curious: If you want to learn how to recite Sanskrit verses, read the section on meter (12.2.1) and listen to some of the audio files listed in Further Resources (12.5).

The Yoga Aficionado: Those familiar already with Kālidāsa's poetry might enjoy the samples of other poetry in 12.2.2.

The Scholar: The Pandit Points in this section have an especially large number of interesting additional readings and discussions of Sanskrit literature (philosophical and literary).

12.1 Vocabulary

Devanāgarī	Transliteration	Part of Speech	Translation
काव्य	kāvya	neut. n.	poetry
चन्द्र	candra	masc. n.	moon
जगत्	jagat	neut. n.	universe, world
नित्य	nitya	adj.	eternal, permanent, fixed
पद	pada	masc. n.	word
परमेश्वर	parameśvara	masc. n., cpd. (*parama* + *īśvara*)	highest lord (Śiva)
पार्वती	pārvatī	fem. n., proper name	Pārvatī (Śiva's wife)
पिता	pitā	masc. sg. nom. n.	father
प्रतिपत्ति	pratipatti	fem. n.	understanding, knowing, acquiring
माता	mātā	fem. sg. nom. n.	mother
मुख	mukha	neut. n.	face
रघुवंश	raghuvaṃśa	masc. n., cpd. (*raghu* + *vaṃśa*)	lineage of Raghu
लोक	loka	masc. n.	world, ordinary people
वन्दे	vande	1 pres. ind. sg. (√*vand*, 1A)	I praise, I honor, I adore, etc.
वाच् (वाग्)	vāc (vāg)	fem. n. (-*g* with sandhi)	speech, language
संपृक्त	saṃpṛkta	ppp. (*sam* + √*pṛc*, 7P)	intermixed, inseparable
संबद्ध	saṃbaddha	ppp. (*sam* + √*badh*, 10P)	tightly connected

12.2 What is Sanskrit Poetry?

KEY POINT: Sanskrit poetry includes a wide range of styles and genres; it has freer word order than prose and understanding meter helps with reading it.

Most of the examples in this book are in prose or verse form, known as श्लोक (*śloka*). That's because, as we have discussed, unlike Sanskrit prose, Sanskrit verse doesn't rely on word order as much to communicate meaning. This use of verse, along with its tendencies toward unusual vocabulary, makes poetry less accessible to the beginner than prose. Poetry in Sanskrit includes what are often called "epics," like the *Rāmāyaṇa* and the *Mahābhārata*.[1] There were also famous collections of "stray verses," or stanzas that may have come from lost, longer poems, or were simply evocative small snippets of poetic imagery.[2] Sanskrit poetry ranged from the erotic to the spiritual, and these two categories are not watertight! The *Śiśupalavadha*, known as a महाकाव्य (*mahākāvya*), or "great poem," has entire sections depicting the god Kṛṣṇa as he engages amorously with beautiful women.[3] Love poetry is also attributed to famous Buddhist philosopher Dharmakīrtī.

The *Raghuvaṃśa*, our example for this lesson, is about the dynasty (*vaṃśa*) of Raghu, whose family includes a long line of famed heroes like Rāma. Not unlike the 1980s soap *Dynasty* and its 2000s-era reboot, the epic poem involves intrigue, violence, and romance. Unlike that soap opera, however, the *Raghuvaṃśa* follows the adventures of

1. Pandit point: Sanskrit dramas were also written in verse form intermixed with prose. Complicating matters, they often included other languages like Prakrit, sometimes characterized as a more vernacular language. For a historical introduction to Prakrit and its relationship to Sanskrit, see Ollett (2017).

2. Pandit point: A stray verse or stanza is known as a सुभाषित (*subhāṣita*).

3. Sections seven through ten of the great poem include these stories. A section or "canto" is called a सर्ग (*sarga*). The entire seventh-century poem is available in English translation in Dundas (2017).

gods—Rāma is a divine incarnation of Viṣṇu, and he ascends to heaven, leaving behind others to manage his kingdom.

We could make a lot of fine-grained distinctions between kinds of poems, but as this book is just an introduction, we'll focus on meter and figures of speech. At this lesson's conclusion, we'll apply these concepts to the opening line of the *Raghuvaṃśa* and part of Mallinātha's commentary.

12.2.1 Kinds of Meter

KEY POINT: Meter in Sanskrit largely depends on the length of vowels. Learning meter is helpful for memorizing and identifying meaningful "chunks" (syntactic units) in verse compositions.

There are now tools for identifying Sanskrit meter online. You can copy and paste a few lines of Sanskrit into a website, hit a button, and it will tell you what meter it's in. While this is a useful tool—and plenty of professionals use such aids—unless you understand something about meter, you can't check for errors. But first, why should you learn about meter, anyway?[4] Why does it matter what a verse's meter is—isn't the goal to just read?

4. Pandit point: Within the Vedic-affirming traditions, one reason to learn meter would be that it's one of the six "limbs" of the Veda (वेदाङ्ग, *vedāṅga*), domains of knowledge that are necessary for understanding and preserving the Veda, although the earliest known text includes both "worldly" or "secular" and Vedic meters. The original text in this discipline is by Piṅgala: the *Chandaḥśāstra* (*Science of Meter*, c. fourth century BCE). However, other groups writing in Sanskrit also found the study of meter and poetry relevant and contributed to poetics. A Jain named Jayadeva wrote his own study of metrics (also called the *Chandaḥśāstra*, about the sixth century CE), though it's mostly a rearrangement of Piṅgala's. And Ratnākaraśānti, who wrote the *Chandoratnākara* (*The Jewel-Treasury of Meter*), and Jñānaśrimitra, who wrote the *Vṛttamālāstuti* (*A Garland of Syllabic Verses for Praise*), were both Buddhists. It's worth noting that these authors are philosophers and poets. See the introduction to Hahn (1982) for a succinct overview of these issues.

Well, no. The goal of Sanskrit poetry is also to hear and recite it. For instance, poetry known as काव्य (*kāvya*) would have been performed in a royal court.[5] The meter is part of the performance, how the poet, the कवि (*kavi*), would have sung the poem. And yes, the poetry was lyrical, sung or chanted (you can hear such chanting in audio recitations online, listed in 12.5 Further Resources at the end of this chapter). So, as you read poetry, reciting is a good idea, and knowing meter helps.

Also, for academics working with multiple versions of a text, understanding meter can help them determine which version might be correct. If we assume that a Sanskrit author is following the rules of meter correctly, then the version where those rules are broken might be rejected as a copyist's error (see Lesson 13 for more on manuscripts and editions). Finally, when it comes to understanding verses, their structure can help identify word boundaries and syntactic units.

Given all these reasons, learning something about meter is essential! As the poetic theorist Daṇḍin says about meter, "For an explorer of the vast ocean depths of poetry, its knowledge is a ship."[6] Let's start assembling our ship, then. We'll work from the smallest parts upward.

Syllables

The basic components of meter are *syllables*.[7] Since the advent of word processors, most of us don't need to know how words divide into syllables. If you type something into a computer, it will automatically insert a hyphen at the right place (usually). The basic idea of a syllable is that it's the word's smallest part. Like Lego blocks that snap together, syllables come together to make words.

---

5. Pandit point: The term काव्य (*kāvya*) has broader and narrower extensions. It can refer to literature generally, including prose and verse compositions. Or it can mean a particular kind of courtly poetry.

6. सा विद्या नौर्विविक्षूणां गम्भीरं काव्यसागरम् ॥ sā vidyā naur vivikṣūṇāṃ gambhīraṃ kāvyasāgaram. *Kāvyadarśa* 1.12.

7. Pandit point: A syllable is an अक्षर (*akṣara*) or a वर्ण (*varṇa*). These two words have different connotations in different contexts, but for our purposes, they're equivalent.

In Sanskrit, the vowel is at the center of a syllable. (By this time, you should know your Sanskrit vowels; if you don't, go back to Lesson 1 for a reminder.) Each vowel counts as a syllable, just by itself, whether long or short. However, vowels often have consonants before them, like क (*ka*). These two sets of sounds have the same number of syllables:

क (*ka*) = 1 syllable
अ (*a*) = 1 syllable

Likewise, sometimes vowels have consonants *after* them. Sometimes, they even have more than one! These sets of sounds also have the same number of syllables:

अन् (*an*) = 1 syllable
निर् (*nir*) = 1 syllable
गच्छ् (*gacch*) = 1 syllable

However, if we add another vowel to each member of this series, we'll add another syllable in nearly every case. That's because each vowel is the center of each syllable. Following Andrew Ollett's notation—see the resources at the end of this lesson—I've shown where a new syllable starts with a period instead of a hyphen since hyphens show divisions between word boundaries.

अक (*a.ka*) = 2 syllables
आ (*ā*) = 1 syllable
अन (*a.na*) = 2 syllables
निर (*ni.ra*) = 2 syllables
गच्छ (*gac.cha*) = 2 syllables

Don't worry about the location of the periods in the last two examples; we'll talk about that next. Do notice, though, that if we strengthen अ (*a*) to आ (*ā*), it remains one syllable.[8] A single vowel, whether long or short,

8. Go back to Lesson 6 if you don't remember the idea of strengthening vowels.

is always a single syllable—that includes diphthongs like ऐ (*ai*). But it is important to pay attention to length—we'll talk about that below.

Words, sentences, and syllables

It should be clear by now that syllables are not words. This is crucial to appreciate in Sanskrit poetry since the patterns that make the verses lyrical depend on syllables.[9] It's not common anymore, but when I was in elementary school, we memorized poetry. The whole class would say the poem in a sing-song voice: "I WANdered LONely AS a CLOUD / That FLOATS on HIGH o'er VALES and hills." It wasn't beautiful, but there was a cadence to the recitation, and it helped us remember the words. Sanskrit poets use something like this in their poetic meters, although it's not quite the same.[10] To appreciate how these meters work, we need to divide words and sentences into syllables. This means we need to learn a few rules about the relationship between consonants and vowels:

1. If a consonant intervenes between two vowels, the consonant (usually) is assigned to the *second* vowel's syllable. From our examples above, which are prefixes:

   निर (*ni.ra*) = 2 syllables

   अन (*a.na*) = 2 syllables

   And examples from complete words:

   इदम् (*i.dam*) = 2 syllables

   निरोध (*ni.ro.dha*) = 3 syllables

9. Pandit point: Strictly speaking, they depend on syllables and on what are called "mora" or मात्र (*mātrā*), which is a unit of weight. Some meters are determined by counting syllables, and some by counting morae. We'll only focus on meters counted by syllable in this book.

10. Pandit point: William Wordsworth's poem is in iambic tetrameter. He uses stress on alternating syllables for his effect. Sanskrit poetry uses length (or "weight") instead. While longer sounds are often also stressed, the two ideas are different.

2. If a consonant conjunct of *two characters* intervenes between vowels, it is split so that the first consonant goes with the first syllable, and the second goes with the second syllable. From our examples above:

   गच्छ (*gac.cha*) = 2 syllables

   And a complete word:

   वाक्य (*vāk.ya*) = 2 syllables

3. If a consonant conjunct with more than *two* consonants intervenes between vowels, the same principle usually applies.[11]

   वात्स्यायन (*vāt.syā.ya.na*) = 4 syllables

   शास्त्र (śās.tra) = 2 syllables

4. If there is an *anusvāra* or *visarga* after a vowel, that is the end of the syllable:

   दुःख (*duḥ.kha*) = 2 syllables

   संस्थिति (*saṃ.sthi.ti*) = 3 syllables

Weights

Now that we know how to divide words into syllables, we have one more step: determining the weight of each syllable. "Weight" really means the length or how long a vowel is held when speaking: heavy syllables are held longer than light syllables.[12] The weight of a syllable depends on the syllable itself as well as the consonants of the syllable that follows it. Below are the basic rules. Syllables are "L" for light and "H" for heavy.

1. **Light:** syllables with short vowels (*a*, *i*, *u*, *ṛ*) are light when they're followed by a syllable starting with a *single* consonant.

   इदम् (*i.dam*) = 2 syllables = L.L

11. Pandit point: If you want to get into the details of these cases, there are rules that depend on the kind of consonant and also situations where consonants are doubled. You can delve into details in the texts listed at the end of the lesson.

12. Pandit point: Heavy syllables are called गुरु (*guru*) and light are लघु (*laghu*).

2. **Heavy:** syllables with long vowels (ā, ī, ū) or diphthongs (*e, ai, o, au*) are heavy. Syllables with short vowels can be heavy when they're followed by *two* consonants, an *anusvāra* (*ṃ*) or *visarga* (*ḥ*).

   दुःख (*duḥ.kha*) = 2 syllables = H.L

   गच्छ (*gac.cha*) = 2 syllables = H.L

Notice that when you put words together, a syllable may become heavy when it was light before. For instance, the syllable *-dam* in the example below changes to heavy if it's followed by a syllable starting with a consonant, like *duḥ-* in *duḥkham.*

इदम् (*i.dam*) = 2 syllables = L.L

इदं दुःख (*i.daṃ.duḥ.kha*) = 4 syllables = L.H.H.L

Meters

Let's look at how these concepts—syllables and weight—combine to make the meter known as *śloka.*[13] Here's a famous example, the opening verse of Kālidāsa's *Raghuvaṃśa*:

वागर्थाविव संपृक्तौ वागर्थप्रतिपत्तये ।
जगतः पितरौ वन्दे पार्वतीपरमेश्वरौ ॥

vāgarthāv iva saṃpṛktau vāgarthapratipattaye |
jagataḥ pitarau vande pārvatīparameśvarau ||

How many syllables are in the first and second lines? Try to count before going on:

vā.gar.thā.vi.va. sam.pṛk.tau. vā.gar.tha.pra.ti.pat.ta.ye |
ja.ga.taḥ. pi.ta.rau. van.de. pār.va.tī.pa.ra.meś.va.rau ||

13. Pandit point: Another term for the *śloka* is अनुष्टुभ् (*anuṣṭubh*), which is the name of a meter according to Piṅgala. But many people use the term *śloka*, including some Sanskrit authors, so we'll stick with it.

We can divide up these two lines—each half of the verse—into equal-size quarters, each called a पाद (*pāda*). We can label the *pādas* with letters to distinguish them:

1a	vā.gar.thā.vi.va. sam.pṛk. tau.	1b	vā.gar.tha.pra.ti.pat.ta.ye
1c	ja.ga.taḥ. pi.ta.rau. van.de.	1d	pār.va.tī.pa.ra.meś.va.rau

Using our rules of heavy and light, we can represent the syllables with "L" and "H":

1a	vā.gar.thā.vi.va. sam.pṛk.tau	1b	vā.gar.tha.pra.ti.pat.ta.ye
1a	H.H.H.L.L.H.H.H	1b	H.H.H.L.L.H.L.H
1c	ja.ga.taḥ. pi.ta.rau. van.de	1d	pār.va.tī.pa.ra.meś.va.rau
1c	L.L.H.L.L.H.H.H	1d	H.L.H.L.L.H.L.H

Now we know roughly how to chant this verse and how long to hold each syllable. But how do we know the meter? There is a pattern for the *śloka* that each of the four quarters must fit. The poet has some choice, though—some syllables could be *either* heavy or light, which I represent with "C."

1a	C.C.C.C.L.H.H.C	1b	C.C.C.C.L.H.L.C
1c	C.C.C.C.L.H.H.C	1d	C.C.C.C.L.H.L.C

Do the quarters match the pattern? Check it out yourself! The pattern itself is pretty simple—three syllables of the first and third quarters, or *pādas* 1a and 1c, must match. Likewise, for the second and fourth quarters, or *pādas* 1b and 1d. (These are marked as either L.H.H or L.H.L above.) All the other syllables are the poet's choice.

Yati/caesura

The last thing you might notice in the example above is that there's a natural split between the first and second and third and fourth quarters, after सम्पृक्तौ (*sampṛktau*) and वन्दे (*vande*). This is the *caesura* in Latin or यति (*yati*) in Sanskrit. It's a break in the verse. Often, these breaks coincide with syntactic units. Having words continue across this break—having a word's syllables or a compound's parts split between the quarters—is typically a poetic flaw, a दोष (*doṣa*), not to be confused with the tasty South Indian rice-flour pancake.[14] As you read verses, paying attention to these segments may help you identify "blocks" of meaning, though this is not a hard-and-fast rule.

12.2.2 Figures of Speech

KEY POINT: There are many figures of speech in Sanskrit, classified according to whether they have to do with sound, meaning, or both. Comparison and punning are two figures of speech involving meaning.

There's an entire discipline devoted to the study of figures of speech. We can distinguish whether a figure of speech depends on the meaning of words or their sound (compare comparison to alliteration), recognize degrees of plausibility in the imagery, identify different grammatical features, and so on. Sanskrit theorists wrote lengthy treatises organizing figures into different categories, like entomologists arranging gorgeous butterflies in display cases. Their purpose was similarly scientific

14. Pandit point: You might wonder if there's an etymological connection between *doṣa* and "dosa," the word for a South Indian food. I could not find scholarly evidence for one, and it seems unlikely, given that Southern India, where the food originates, would have used Dravidian languages like Tamil. However, there's an enjoyable (though almost certainly false) folk etymology about the term. Supposedly, long ago, a brahman tried to make alcohol from fermented rice. His home-brew experiment was a failure, but the resulting batter made a nice thin pancake. Since the original source—alcohol—was against his ethical precepts, the dish was a "flaw" or a "sin," a दोष (*doṣa*) in Sanskrit.

and philosophical in the same way, but they also wanted skillful audiences to appreciate the beauty of poetry. Below, we'll look at two of the specimens that these thinkers observed and analyzed:

Comparison (*upamā, rūpaka*)

Comparison is the heart of poetry.[15] In English rhetoric, we'd call this sentence a *metaphor* since it identifies two things that are not, strictly speaking, the same: an abstract idea like comparison is not a physical organ. In Sanskrit poetics, रूपक (*rūpaka*) is the term for figures of speech that imaginatively identify two different things. Were I to say instead, "Comparison is *like* the heart of poetry," this would be a *simile* since it is more comparison than identification. This is उपमा (*upamā*).[16]

A very common term used to compare two words is इव (*iva*), meaning "like." As we saw in Lesson 9, when reading sentences with this term, it's important to know what is being compared to what. Comparing love to a flower is one thing (love is beautiful, it blossoms . . .), but comparing a flower to love is another (a flower is an abstract concept?). Sanskrit aesthetic theorists laid out plenty of grammatical and aesthetic

---

15. For a nice introduction to comparison in the work of Daṇḍin, see Bronner (2007). An encyclopedic treatment of figures of speech is available in Gerow (1971). Bronner (2007, 93) nicely translates Appaya Dīkṣita's verse, which recursively engages in comparison while discussing it:

Simile is the sole actress on the stage of poetry,
and yet she performs a vast variety of roles.
When she dances
she captivates the hearts
of those who know her secret.

उपमैका शैलुसी सम्प्राप्ता चित्रभूमिकाभेदान् । रञ्जयति काव्यरङ्गे नृत्यन्ती तद्विदां चेतः ॥
upamaikā śailusī samprāptā citrabhūmikābhedān | rañjayati kāvyaraṅge nṛtyantī tadvidāṃ cetaḥ ||

16. Pandit point: Trying to map English and Sanskrit terms for figures of speech is a challenge. Not every *upamā* has a comparative term like English similes do. Sanskrit theorists carved up the conceptual territory differently. See Gerow's (1971) introduction to his wide-ranging *Glossary* for discussion.

requirements for making comparisons, though they are difficult to encapsulate. Sometimes comparisons can involve words with different grammatical genders (a masculine noun compared to a feminine noun), but other times, they shouldn't. For our purposes, we can identify several different comparative strategies:

1. Using comparative terms (*yathā*, *iva*)

   A is like B.

   यथा चन्द्रस्तथा मुखम् ।

   yathā candras tathā mukham.

   Like the moon, so the face.

   चन्द्र इव मुखम ।

   candra iva mukham.

   The face is like the moon.

2. Using a nominal ending (*-vat*)

   A is B-like.

   मुखश्चन्द्रवत् ।

   mukhaś candravat.

   The face is moon-like.

3. Using a compound

   B-A.

   चन्द्रमुखः ।

   candramukhaḥ.

   He has a moon-face.

4. Suggesting comparisons through indirect means

   तस्याश्चेन्मुखमस्ति सौम्यसुभगं किं पार्वेणेनदुना ।

   tasyāś cen mukham asti saumyasubhagaṃ kiṃ pārveṇenadunā.

> When we have the fair clarity of her face, who would care for the full-orbed moon?[17]
>
> (This line implicitly compares a face to a moon.)

When reading Sanskrit poetry (and Sanskrit literature in general), be on the lookout for comparisons, explicit or implicit.

Bitextual meanings (*śleṣa*)

When isn't a door a door? When it's ajar! That pun usually provokes groans, not poetic beauty. In English, puns are typically bad jokes. But in Sanskrit, puns, or double meanings known as श्लेष (*śleṣa*), are one of the many tools that a poet has at their disposal for evocative writing.[18] In fact, because of how many meanings a single word can have in Sanskrit, combined with the rules of sandhi, some Sanskrit poems can be read in two or more ways. There's a famous poem which, when read forward, tells the story of the *Mahābhārata*, and read backward, the *Rāmāyaṇa*. Now that's *extreme* poetry.[19] The famous literary theorist Ānandavardhana quotes an example of *śleṣa* from Harṣadeva's *Ratnāvalī* (*Jewel-necklace*) 2.4, and his commentator helps us out by explaining how the verses work. The phrases with double meanings are in italics:[20]

17. Translation of Vāmana's *Kāvyālaṃkāra* from Ingalls, Masson, and Patwardhan (1990, 143). Sanskrit (GRETIL): तस्याश्चेन्मुखमस्ति सौम्यसुभगं किं पार्वेणेनदुना । *tasyāś cen mukham asti saumyasubhagaṃ kiṃ pārveṇenadunā*. For the construction *kim* + instrumental, an unpoetic but memorable trick (for TV-watchers of a certain age) is to call it the "Seinfeld construction." Just imagine Jerry Seinfeld saying, arms outstretched, "What's the deal with . . . ?" This construction asks what (*kim*) is the purpose for (instrumental) a noun. (I owe this lively analogy to Matthew Dasti.)

18. Pandit point: The gender-neutral pronoun "their" is intentional. While much Sanskrit poetry is written by men, there were women writing poetry as well. See Pal (2010), for instance.

19. Pandit point: For this (*Rāghavayādavīya*) and other poems that use this kind of double (or more!) meaning, see the aptly titled *Extreme Poetry*, Bronner (2010).

20. Translation adapted from Ingalls, Masson, and Patwardhan (1990, 278–79).

Reading 1:

It is bursting with *new buds* and is pallid, *it* has just begun to *blossom*

It responds (*swayingly*) to *the constant breezes*:

this garden vine today *on its madana tree*

is like a rival woman, and by my gazing on it

I shall doubtless make my queen's face flush with anger.

Reading 2:

She is bursting with *longing* and is pallid, *she* has just begun to *stretch her limbs*

She responds (*feverishly*) to *her constant sighs*.

This garden vine today *in her passion*

is like a rival woman, and by my gazing on it

I shall doubtless make my queen's face flush with anger.[21]

Since the word for garden (*adyodyāna-*) vine (*-latā*) is grammatically feminine, Harṣadeva can play with this ambiguity, making adjectives modifying that word refer to a woman. New buds or longing (*utkālikā*) can both "burst" or appear suddenly. Women in love are supposed to yawn and stretch their limbs (*jṛmbhā*), but this word also can mean "opening" or "expanding," like when flowers blossom. There's a tree called the *madana*, and a vine can be "with" or "on" that tree by affixing *sa-* in compound. But *madana* also means "intoxicating" or being overwhelmed by love. The play on words here isn't coincidental, either—there is a comparison between the woman and the vine, making this an

21. उद्दामोत्कलिकां विपाण्डुररुचं प्रारब्धजृम्भां क्षणादायासं श्वसनोद्गमैरविरतैरातन्वतीमात्मनः ।
अद्योद्यानलतामिमां समदनां नारीमिवान्यां ध्रुवं पश्यन्कोपविपाटलद्युति मखं देव्याः करिष्याम्यहम् ।।

uddāmotkalikāṃ vipāṇḍurarucaṃ prārabdhajṛmbhāṃ
kṣaṇād āyāsaṃ śvasanodgamair aviratair ātanvatīm ātmanaḥ |
adyodyānalatām imāṃ samadanāṃ nārīm ivānyāṃ
dhruvaṃ paśyan kopavipāṭaladyuti mukhaṃ devyāḥ kariṣyāmy aham ||

उपमाश्लेष (*upamāśleṣa*). This compound term means a pun (*śleṣa*) that is a comparison (*upamā*). In other words, the double meanings of the words aren't just any arbitrary meanings but form a comparison. And it's a common one: Sanskrit poets often compare beautiful women with slender arms and light skin to fragile vines with pale flowers.

Unlike straightforward comparisons, there are no easy tricks to identify and understand श्लेष (*śleṣa*). But your new understanding of the grammar and lexicon of Sanskrit will help you appreciate it when you encounter it in translations (often in footnotes since it's nearly impossible to capture in a single translation). And, if you read poetry, you are now attuned to how poets use ambiguity to their advantage. While there are many more—perhaps innumerable—figures of speech in Sanskrit poetry, these two will give you a start in appreciating its riches.

12.3 Putting Everything Together

वागर्थाविव संपृक्तौ वागर्थप्रतिपत्तये ।

जगतः पितरौ वन्दे पार्वतीपरमेश्वरौ ॥ १।१

वागर्थाविव शब्दार्थाविव संपृक्तौ नित्यसंबद्धावित्यर्थः ।
जगतो लोकस्य पितरौ। माता च पिता च पितरौ । पार्वती च
परमेश्वरशश्च पार्वतीपरमेश्वरौ ।

vāgarthāv iva samprktau vāgarthapratipattaye |

jagataḥ pitarau vande pārvatīparameśvarau || 1.1

vāgarthāv iva śabdārthāv iva saṃpṛktau nityasaṃbaddhāv
ity arthaḥ. jagato lokasya pitarau. mātā ca pitā ca pitarau.
pārvatī ca parameśvaraśaś ca pārvatīparameśvarau.

The reading for this lesson includes the opening verse of the *Raghuvaṃśa*, the poet Kālidāsa's prayer to the Lord Parameśvara and his consort,

Pārvatī, to help him with his composition. It's a famous *śloka*, not only for its use in the *Raghuvaṃśa* but also later adaptations—even up to the present day.[22] The verse is within a commentarial reading from the *Saṃjīvanī* by Mallinātha (late fourteenth to fifteenth century CE). Mallinātha is a well-known commentator who wrote not only on Kālidāsa's poetry but also the epically long महाकाव्य (*mahākāvya*) mentioned earlier. In his remarks on the first verse of the *Raghuvaṃśa,* he helps readers parse which words are separate and which are in compounds. He also gives us analyses of the compounds.[23]

How two things are connected (*saṃpṛkta*) is like वागर्थ (*vāgartha*). And what does this compound mean? Mallinātha glosses it with a synonym: शब्दार्थाविव (*śabdārthāv iva*). So we should understand वाग् (*vāg*) as equivalent to speech (*śabda*), and the two things connected are like that.[24] And what about संपृक्तौ (*saṃpṛktau*) itself? He says that it is "permanently related" (*nityasaṃbaddhāv*). Having glossed these terms, he concludes with the phrase we now recognize from Lesson 11: "this is the meaning" (*ity arthaḥ*).[25]

---

22. For instance, this line opens a famous song by Ilaiyaraaja. He is one of the most esteemed Indian composers in the modern day and wrote it for a 1983 Tamil film, *Sagara Sangamam*. (Thanks to Suresh Kumar for pointing this out.)

23. Pandit point: While we have talked about "commentaries" as if they are one unified genre, there are many differences among commentaries, depending on the kind of root text they're working with and the particular goal of the commentary. Patel (2022) is a nice (albeit scholarly) discussion of the particularities of commentaries on Sanskrit literature, *kāvya*. In summary, Patel says that these kinds of commentaries "teach the *skill* of reading" but don't aim to give a particular reading (2022, 14). Still, Mallinātha is known for being polemical about his interpretations being better than others, to the extent that today, there's a saying that stubbornly holding onto one's own ideas is "doing a Mallināthi (*mallināthī-karaṇam*)" (Patel 2014, 62–63).

24. Pandit point: The word वाग् (*vāg*) is originally वाच् (*vāc*) but with final-consonant sandhi. See Lesson 7.

25. Pandit point: In a section I've excluded from the excerpt, Mallinātha goes on to talk about what this phrase means, appealing to philosophers in a tradition known as "Mīmāṃsā." Mīmāṃsā philosophers argue that words cannot acquire their meanings conventionally at a certain point in time, but rather, they must have always had the

Each successive sentence analyzes or glosses the next part of the verse. The only word Mallinātha does not explain is वन्दे (*vande*), the first person singular of the verb √वन्द् (1A), which we haven't learned in this book.

वागर्थाविव संपृक्तौ वागर्थप्रतिपत्तये ।
जगतः पितरौ वन्दे पार्वतीपरमेश्वरौ ॥ १।१

vāgarthāv iva saṃpṛktau vāgarthapratipattaye |
jagataḥ pitarau vande pārvatīparameśvarau || 1.1

Here's how this verse would be translated, very literally, with each *pāda* in turn:

> To those two who, like speech and meaning (*vāgarthāv iva*) are interconnected (*saṃpṛktau*),
>
> for my goal of understanding speech and meaning (*vāgarthapratipattaye*),
>
> I give praise (*vande*) to the universe's two parents (*jagataḥ pitarau*),[26]
>
> Pārvatī-Parameśvara (*pārvatīparameśvarau*).

Because of the case-declined nature of Sanskrit, from the very beginning, we know the verse is about *two things*, which are an object of some action—because we have a dual accusative (*saṃpṛktau*). We get to the verb, *vande*, only in the third quarter, and the focal point of the verse

meaning-referent relationship. This reference exemplifies how philosophy and poetry are interwoven in Sanskrit literature. Grammar, too—Mallinātha cites Pāṇini and Patañjali in his commentary, which most poetic commentators do.

26. Pandit point: The masculine noun पितृ (*pitṛ*) in the singular means "father," but in the dual, means "parents," which includes both father and mother. The declension for this kind of noun, ending in -तृ (*-tṛ*), is one of many we will not get to in detail in this book. But by now, you can probably recognize that in this form, the vocalic ऋ (*ṛ*) strengthens to अर् (*ar*) before an ending is applied. This declension is one of the few places where the long ॠ (*ṝ*) appears in the accusative plural पितॄन् (*pitṝn*) and genitive plural पितॄणाम् (*pitṝṇām*).

arrives at the end. See if you can work out the rest of the commentary on your own.

12.4 About the Reading: Sound and Meaning, Pārvatī and Śiva

While much of Mallinātha's commentary on the opening of the *Raghuvaṃśa* is fairly basic compound analysis, he does explain the relationship between speech or sound (*śabda*) as being "eternal" or "permanent" (*nitya*). Further, the relationship between Pārvatī and Śiva is also supposed to be *nitya*, but there are many stories explaining how they met. What is going on?

First of all, although Kālidāsa narrates stories of Pārvatī and Śiva meeting and falling in love, there is a sense in which both of these gods are beyond time—not only are there stories of Pārvatī being married to Śiva in past lives, then reincarnating to be married to him again, but the goddess herself is, in many traditions, understood as feminine energy itself (and Śiva, masculine energy). So, their pairing is a cosmological reality beyond just a single couple.

As for the claim that sound and meaning are paired like these two deities, this is a view found in Mīmāṃsā (roughly translatable as "hermeneutics"). According to Mīmāṃsakas ("hermeneuticists"), sound must be paired with meanings in a permanent manner to avoid arbitrariness. If human beings could pair any sound with any meaning—that is, if we could individually cause a beginning to the speech-meaning relationship—then there would be no communication. Just imagine if each of us had our own personal sounds that we connected (somehow!) to meanings. No one would understand each other. At least, something like this is the basic idea behind the claim that the relationship between meaningful sounds and their referents must have existed long, long before human speakers. For more on this topic, see Taber (1989, 2016). On Śiva and Pārvatī, see Kramrisch (1992) and Tubb (1984).

12.5 Further Resources

A clear online introduction to meters is found on Andrew Ollett's "Sanskrit at UChicago" website, which includes helpful videos, audio, and diagrams.

Ollett, Andrew. n.d. "Meters: A Guide to Sanskrit and Prakrit Meters." Sanskrit at UChicago. http://prakrit.info/vrddhi/meter/.

The appendix to Apte's dictionary includes a discussion of meters:

Apte, V. S. 1957–1959. *The Practical Sanskrit–English Dictionary.* Poona: Prasad Prakashan.

For identifying meters, two "Sanskrit metres" websites are handy:

Shreevatsa. n.d. "Sanskrit Metres." Accessed October 23, 2022. https://sanskritmetres.appspot.com/.

Terdalkar, Hrishikesh. n.d. "Chandojñānam." Jñānasaṅgrahaḥ. Accessed October 23, 2022. https://sanskrit.iitk.ac.in/jnanasangraha/chanda/.

For a more thorough treatment than the above, which is written accessibly, see:

Morgan, Les B. 2011. *Croaking Frogs: A Guide to Sanskrit Metrics and Figures of Speech*. Mahodara Press. Accompanying website with audio files: www.mywhatever.com/sanskrit/frogs.

On reading South Asian (not just Sanskrit) literature in translation, including discussions and examples of Sanskrit poetry:

Bronner, Yigal, and Charles Hallisey. 2022. *Sensitive Reading. University of California Press*. University of California Press. https://doi.org/10.1525/luminos.114.

V. M. Kale's English translation of the *Raghuvaṃśa* includes the Sanskrit and Mallinātha's commentary, making it a good text to practice with:

Kale, V. M. 1957. *The Raghuvaṃśa of Kālidāsa*. 5th ed. Delhi: Motilal Banarsidass.

For a longer treatment, an older guide to Sanskrit meter by Charles Philip Brown is in the public domain and available freely online through the Hathi Trust:

Brown, Charles Philip. 1869. *Sanskrit Prosody and Numerical Symbols Explained*. London: Trübner & Co. https://catalog.hathitrust.org/Record/011608715.

Self-Quiz Answer

Answer: there are sixteen syllables.

Lesson 13

Reading: Bhagavadgītā 3.14–15

अन्नाद्भवन्ति भूतानि पर्जन्यादन्नसंभवः ।
यज्ञाद्भवति पर्जन्यो यज्ञः कर्मसमुद्भवः
॥१४॥

कर्म ब्रह्मोद्भवं विद्धि ब्रह्माक्षरसमुद्भवम् ।
तस्मात्सर्वगतं ब्रह्म नित्यं यज्ञे प्रतिष्ठितम्
॥१५॥

annād bhavanti bhūtāni parjanyād
annasaṃbhavaḥ |
yajñād bhavati parjanyo yajñaḥ
karmasamudbhavaḥ ||14
karma brahmodbhavaṃ viddhi
brahmākṣarasamudbhavam |
tasmāt sarvagataṃ brahma nityaṃ yajñe
pratiṣṭhitam ||15

Points of Interest For

The Curious: You can skip 13.2.3 if you don't plan to work with lots of editions, but do read 13.2.1 to understand different kinds of translations.

The Yoga Aficionado: Read 13.2.4 on comparing translations—perhaps pick out some of your favorite translations of a text to look at afterwards.

The Scholar: If you plan to engage with critical editions, don't skip 13.2.3.

13.1 Vocabulary

Devanāgarī	Transliteration	Part of Speech	Translation
अक्षर	akṣara	neut. n.	a syllable; the syllable *om* (ॐ)
अन्न	anna	neut. n.	food; rice
उद्	ud	pfx.	out of, from (with verb bhū)
नित्य	nitya	adj.	eternal, permanent
पर्जन्य	parjanya	masc. n. (or proper name)	rain; Parjanya god of rain
भव (+ सम्, + उद्)	bhava (+ sam, + ud)	masc. n.	coming into existence, production, origin.
भूत	bhūta	adj. (ppp. from √भू, 1P)	lit., what has become; being
यज्ञ	yajña	masc. n.	offering, sacrifice; worship, devotion
विद्धि	viddhi	2 sg. impv. from √विद् (2P)	you, know!
सम्	sam	pfx.	together, along with
सर्व	sarva	adj.	all, every

13.2 Lesson Overview

KEY POINT: Sanskrit translations can differ significantly, so learning how to read and compare them is essential.

The *Bhagavadgītā,* part of the *Mahābhārata*, is one of the most translated texts of all time. Chances are, if you want to learn Sanskrit, being able to read the *Gītā*, as it's often called for short, is part of your motivation. This part of the *Mahābhārata* tells the story of the Pāṇḍava prince, Arjuna, who is about to engage in battle but stops, overcome with agony when he sees friends, family, and former teachers lined up across from him. He must kill them—mustn't he? His friend and cousin Kṛṣṇa—who is also a god incarnate, Viṣṇu—gives him advice, helping him to understand why he *must* fight and what his place is in the great cosmic cycle of life, death, and rebirth.

In this lesson, we'll focus on how to approach reading a Sanskrit text like the *Gītā* along with translations. If translations differ, is it possible to know what the text "really means"? What tools should you use to understand why translators differ? What should you look for when reading, now that you know some Sanskrit?

13.2.1 Kinds of Translations

KEY POINT: Since translations differ in the materials they rely on, it is important to read a translation's introduction to determine what kind of edition the translator is using.

Perhaps you've had this experience: you brought a bottle of bubbly wine to a party, and the host took it gingerly, with a bit of a raised eyebrow: "You know, it's not *really* champagne unless it's from the Champagne region of France." The imprimatur of "champagne" in France is very particular. But whether your party gift was sparkling wine or actual champagne, it probably tasted just fine and had the desired effects. When it comes to Sanskrit translations, there are translations, and then there are translations. It's important to know that not all translations are made from the same kinds of materials, just like not all sparkling wine comes from the Champagne region of France. However, depending on your aims, this may not matter.

A brief stage-setting: Sanskrit texts in the subcontinent were traditionally written on palm leaves bound together in the center with string to make long, rectangular books, as in Figure 4.

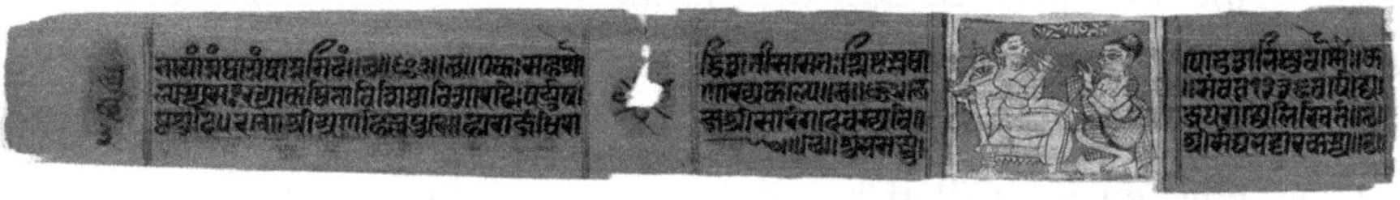

Figure 4. Image of a Jain manuscript, the *Kalpasūtra*, from the Cleveland Museum of Art

These texts were very fragile in the heat and humidity of the Indian subcontinent and had to be recopied every hundred years or so to preserve the material. As you might imagine, scribes who copied these texts occasionally made mistakes. The books were transported around the region, and over time, different versions came about.

While these differences are often minor, sometimes they can be significant, especially for widely disseminated and very ancient orally transmitted texts, like the *Mahābhārata*, which exists in different regional versions or "recensions."[1] Even before the modern science of text criticism—the practice of reconstructing an original version of a text based on variations—Sanskrit commentators would identify and correct what they thought were misreadings.[2] Today, many palm-leaf

1. Pandit point: With a text like the *Mahābhārata*, as the authors of the critical edition note, there is no single original written text that such an edition is restoring. That's because it spread orally as well as through written versions. Part of the text's history is this organic process of people adding and redacting the lengthy story. See Mehendale (2007) for some scholarly discussion of this point. A more accessible discussion is found in Doniger (2009).

2. Pandit point: Pollock (2015) discusses some examples of the editing practices in Sanskrit. He quotes the sixteenth-century commentator Vādirāja as saying, "Many thousands of manuscripts have disappeared, and those that are extant have become disordered. So confused can a text have become that even the gods themselves could not figure it out" (120). But even earlier, in the tenth century, we see commentators on *kāvya*, such as Vallabhadeva having to decide which reading—that is, which manuscript's version—makes the most sense in different places (121). This isn't to say premodern Sanskrit textual work is like modern textual criticism. Pollock's article explains many points of difference.

manuscripts form the basis for printed Sanskrit editions, typeset in modern scripts like (but not only) Devanāgarī. Now, philologists and Indologists work to date and compare different versions of texts, both manuscripts and printed editions, to identify the best-unified text they can reconstruct, with lots of footnotes indicating where different editions diverge.

These editions are called "critical editions" and represent the sustained work of scholars. Let's return to our sparkling wine and champagne analogy. Just like when buying fancy wine, when looking at a translation, one of the first things to do is determine the source. Was the translation made from a critical edition systematically collecting many manuscripts and editions? Was it made from a single printed edition or manuscript? From the translator's own choices among what they thought made sense? The differences here are subtle, not entirely unlike the difference between the origins of wines.[3] After all, critical editions take decades or longer, and there's also nothing inherently wrong with a translation based on a single edition (as long as that's made clear). However, by looking at the source of your translation, you can compare it with other translations in an informed manner. If two translations use different sources, you might be comparing apples and oranges—or Champagne and California grapes.[4] So, read the introduction to your translation. A serious translator will

3. As with all analogies, there are limitations, of course! It's illegal to label something "Champagne" if it isn't made from certain kinds of grapes in certain regions. But translations from noncritical editions are still *translations*. At the same time, unlike wine, where we might say there's a lot of subjectivity in whether wine is good, there are some objective criteria for when a translation has gotten things right and when an edition is better than another. However, as Sanskrit philosophers have pointed out in their discussion of fallacies known as *samas*, two objects do not need to be the same in order to be usefully compared.

4. Some translations of Sanskrit texts will also be from other languages, like Chinese and Tibetan. This is especially true for Buddhist texts, which traveled widely throughout Asia. Occasionally, we have portions in Chinese, portions in Tibetan, and a few fragments in Sanskrit. There is also a practice of "back-translating" Tibetan translations of lost Sanskrit texts into Sanskrit because these translators were known for being very systematic in their approaches. Sometimes, such texts have been found later and shown to match these back-translations very closely!

identify their sources. (If they don't, be skeptical—they may be "translating" by putting another translation in their own words.)

13.2.2 Translation Conventions

KEY POINT: To fully understand a translation and its relationship to the Sanskrit text, it is crucial to understand what brackets, parentheses, and hyphens mean.

Translators and publishing companies vary, so it is always important to look at the introductory material to the translation you're reading for specifics about that particular version. However, there are a few conventions that are widely shared.

Bracket types

Typically, translators will use square brackets [ ] to insert words which, while not strictly in the Sanskrit, are strongly implied or necessitated by the syntax. For instance, sometimes they will replace a pronoun with its referent this way:

> स गच्छति (*sa gacchati*)
> *Literal:* He goes.
> *Bracketed*: [The king] goes.

You will also see round parentheses ( ) to insert explanatory remarks. Typically, these words aren't suggested by the syntax but are to help readers understand the meaning. The sentence above, then, could be further expanded:

> स गच्छति (*sa gacchati*)
> *Literal:* He goes.
> *Bracketed*: [The king] goes.
> *Bracketed and parenthetical*: [The king] goes (to the court).

The difference between the brackets and parentheses allows you to recognize what is more directly related to the text and what is more interpretive. In context, the pronoun needs a referent—although in some texts, that referent may be more complicated to determine than others. But note that there is no object for "goes" in the Sanskrit sentence—the translation adds it in parentheses for clarity.

Transliterations

You have learned how to transliterate into Roman script from Devanāgarī using what is known as IAST, the International Alphabet of Sanskrit Transliteration. This is a very standard, widely used system. However, there are different transliteration styles using this same system. They differ in particular with how they treat boundaries between words in compounds. Take our very first Sanskrit compound, in Lesson 2, which we transliterated this way:

> योगश्चित्तवृत्तिनिरोधः
> yogaś cittavṛttinirodhaḥ

Authors will often use this approach, which lacks any hyphens inside the compound *cittavṛttinirodhaḥ*. It's especially common in academic journals intended for Sanskritists. But you will also commonly see:

> योगश्चित्तवृत्तिनिरोधः
> yogaś citta-vṛtti-nirodhaḥ

In this system, the transliteration includes hyphens within compounds at the boundaries between words. This can be helpful since, as we have learned, there may be several ways to disambiguate sandhi. Essentially the translator is saying, "This is how *I* read the Sanskrit." They are showing their work. But you will also see variations on this theme, which we must illustrate by looking at a compound with sandhi:

> वाक्यार्थः
> vākyārthaḥ

In this compound, the transliteration does not put a hyphen between the two words, *vākya* and *artha*, because the two vowels merge through sandhi. As a reader now aware of sandhi rules, it's up to you to recognize that these are *two* words. Another strategy makes this a bit easier:

वाक्यार्थः
vākyârthaḥ

Notice the little mark on top of the "a." The symbol ^ is called a circumflex. It is equivalent to the macron ¯ in one sense: it means the Sanskrit vowel is long. (In Sanskrit transliteration, you will only see this symbol over vowels.) However, it differs from the macron, since it indicates that the vowel is a result of sandhi. This signals that the *â* can be disambiguated in several ways (quick pop quiz: What are they? go back to Lesson 4 to remind yourself).[5]

13.2.3 Reading Critical Editions

> **KEY POINT:** A critical edition uses a notation system to identify the different manuscripts and printed editions from which the editor has reconstructed a single text.

Suppose you have a critical edition of a Sanskrit text that you'd like to look at along with a translation. How should you begin? Reading the introduction is the first step, as we've noted. This will prepare you for the system of transliteration and notation that the translator and editor use. Figure 5 presents a critical edition that you might encounter for a verse of the *Bhagavadgītā*.[6]

5. Pandit point: There is yet another system of transliteration used mostly by the Clay Sanskrit Library. They explain it in the introductions to their books: their system replaces the usual hyphen, the -, with a vertical bar |. Their approach to sandhi across word boundaries is more complex for metrical reasons. Instead of *vākyârthaḥ*, you might see *vaky'|ârthaḥ*.

6. I have recreated this based on Belvalkar (1968).

अन्नाद्भवन्ति भूतानि पर्जन्यादन्नसंभवः ।

यज्ञाद्भवति पर्जन्यो यज्ञः कर्मसमुद्भवः ॥१४॥

---

14. [c]) G_3 धर्माद्; $C_{\bar{a}, g, k, l, m, n, r, \acute{s}, u}$ यज्ञाद् (as in text).
– [d]) $\acute{S}_1$, $K_{1, 2}$, $\tilde{\acute{N}}_1$, D_{a1} यज्ञ-; $C_{\bar{a}, k, l, n, r, \acute{s}, u}$ यज्ञः (as in text).

Figure 5. Sample critical edition, *Bhagavadgītā* 3.14

As we learned in Lesson 12, a verse quarter (*pāda*) is often identified by letters: "a," "b," "c," and "d." Here, the editor has identified two variant readings and which parts of the verse they correspond to: c) or d). After each *pāda* letter, capital letters identify manuscripts and editions. To know precisely what these letters mean, we must look in the introduction. Here are two examples from the third *pāda*, c):

> G_3 = Pudukotah, State Library, No 260.
>
> $C_{\bar{a}}$ = Ānandavardhana's commentary, the *Jñānakarmasamuccaya*, Bombay Govt. Collection (BORI), manuscript no. 179 of 1883–84.

The first is a manuscript of the *Mahābhārata*, found as a physical copy in a library. The second is a commentary on the *Mahābhārata*, also in manuscript form. Because the commentator would have been working with a certain version of the text, these variants tell us what versions were like at that time. For two words, there are two alternate readings, which we can identify by comparing the one "as in the text" with the other reading, identified by where it was found. You can look at Figure 6 to see the two readings circled.

अन्नाद्भवन्ति भूतानि पर्जन्यादन्नसंभवः ।

यज्ञाद्भवति पर्जन्यो यज्ञः कर्मसमुद्भवः ॥१४॥

---

14. c) G_3 धर्माद्; $C_{\bar{a}, g, k, l, m, n, r, \acute{s}, u}$ यज्ञाद् (as in text).
– d) $\acute{S}_1$, $K_{1, 2}$, $\tilde{\acute{N}}_1$, D_{a1} यज्ञ-; $C_{\bar{a}, k, l, n, r, \acute{s}, u}$ यज्ञः (as in text).

Figure 6. Sample critical edition with annotations, *Bhagavadgītā* 3.14

Here's how the second line of this verse would look, with the reading according to manuscript G_3 in bold:

> धर्माद्भवति पर्जन्यो यज्ञः कर्मसमुद्भवः
> **dharmād** bhavati parjanyo yajñaḥ karmasamudbhavaḥ[7]

Now, try to reproduce what the second line of the verse would look like according to $\acute{S}_1$ and the other variants. Hint: notice that there is a hyphen in the variant यज्ञ- (*yajña-*). (Answer at the end of the lesson.) The ability to read a critical edition allows you to identify the sources of different translations. And, if you want to read scholarly writing about Sanskrit, academics will often refer to critical editions.

13.2.4 Comparing Translations

> **KEY POINTS:** As you compare translations, pay attention not only to different translations of single words but also to other details, such as whether the text is in prose or verse, how clauses are ordered, and whether sentences are split differently.

7. Pandit point: Remember that, unlike printed Devanāgarī, Roman transliterations will often split conjuncts, which happen at word boundaries, like the -द्भ (*-dbh*) in धर्माद्भवति (*dharmād-bhavati*). Editions and transliterations can have mistakes and inconsistencies, however, so keep an eye out. Just because words are combined doesn't guarantee they are in compound. And, as we've seen, vowel sandhi is not split in transliteration, even if it joins two different words.

In the last part of this lesson, we'll look at several different translations of the verse we just saw printed in the critical edition. The goal is for you to reflect on questions to ask as you read Sanskrit translations. Here are the verses again:

> अन्नाद्भवन्ति भूतानि पर्जन्यादन्नसंभवः ।
> यज्ञाद्भवति पर्जन्यो यज्ञः कर्मसमुद्भवः ॥१४॥
> कर्म ब्रह्मोद्भवं विद्धि ब्रह्माक्षरसमुद्भवम् ।
> तस्मात्सर्वगतं ब्रह्म नित्यं यज्ञे प्रतिष्ठितम् ॥१५॥
> annād bhavanti bhūtāni parjanyād annasaṃbhavaḥ |
> yajñād bhavati parjanyo yajñaḥ karmasamudbhavaḥ ||14
> karma brahmodbhavaṃ viddhi brahmākṣarasamudbhavam |
> tasmāt sarvagataṃ brahma nityaṃ yajñe pratiṣṭhitam ||15

Below are several translations of the verses. Read them and jot down what you notice. Where do they agree and where do they disagree? What different choices have they made?[8] As you read, identify which words and phrases in Sanskrit correspond to the English translations. Some notes to help: one important pattern is a sequence of ablatives like अन्नात् (*annāt*), which expresses the origin of different things (in the nominative case), where the verbal element is various forms of √भू (*bhū*). I've given you the imperative form विद्धि (*viddhi*) in the vocabulary list—like the optative mood, this verb mood has a particular force. It is a command, conjugated here in the second person singular, so it is addressed to the hearer (in the text, this is Arjuna, listening to Kṛṣṇa).

1. From food creatures come into being; from rain food is produced, from sacrifice comes rain, and sacrifice is born of action. (14) Know that (ritual) action arises from Brahman (the Veda), and that Brahman arises from the Imperishable. Therefore,

8. For two articles discussing translation choices on these passages in the *Bhagavadgītā* in more detail, see Larson (1981) and Keating (2019).

Brahman, the all pervading, is ever established in sacrifice. (15)[9]

2. Creatures depend on food,
food comes from rain,
rain depends on sacrifice,
and sacrifice comes from action. (14)
Action comes from the spirit of prayer,
whose source is OM,[10] sound of the imperishable;
so the pervading infinite spirit
is ever present in rites of sacrifice. (15)[11]

3. Beings exist
through food.
Parjanya, the rain,
is the source of food.
Parjanya exists
through sacrifice
and sacrifice
exists through action. (14)
Know the origin
of sacrificial action
as Brahman,
arising from
the eternal nature
of Brahman;
thus all-pervading Brahman
is eternally fixed
in sacrifice. (15)[12]

9. Deutsch (1968, 49).

10. Pandit point: The sound "OM" (also symbolized as ॐ and transliterated as *oṃ*) is linked with the idea of Sanskrit and India in popular media. It's a syllable that is part of ancient Vedic ritual, theorized variously by philosophical traditions—though typically deeply connected with creation, emergence, and power. As it's a syllable, the word for syllable, अक्षर (*akṣara*), evokes it specifically in many contexts. But अक्षर (*akṣara*) as an adjective also simply means "imperishable."

11. Stoler-Miller (1986, 45).

12. Patton (2008, 39).

4. Living creatures are nourished by food, and food is nourished by rain; rain itself is the water of life, which comes from selfless worship and service. (14)
   Every selfless act, Arjuna, is born from Brahman, the eternal, infinite Godhead. Brahman is present in every act of service. (15)[13]

Comparing these translations, you will notice several differences. Some translations represent the Sanskrit in a kind of verse format (2, 3). Others simply present each verse in a separate sentence (1, 4). Word choices are different, especially for पर्जन्य (*parjanya*), यज्ञ (*yajña*), कर्मन् (*karman*), and ब्रह्मन् (*brahman*). That difficult concept, *brahman*, which we saw in Lesson 4 and Lesson 6, is translated as "infinite spirit" (2), left as "Brahman" (1, 3), or translated as "Brahman" and glossed as "Godhead" (4). Even an apparently simple word like *karman* is treated differently: a parenthetical insertion in (1) suggests it is a restricted kind of action, "(ritual) action," whereas (3) inserts "sacrificial" before "action" but without the parentheses. The last version (4) uses a phrase to fill out the translator's interpretation of the word: "selfless worship and service" in verse 14 and "selfless act" in 15.

If you read only one of these translations, you might come away with a very different understanding of the text than if you read another. You are now in a position to look at several translations and ask yourself what choices the translators have made. You also can look at commentaries to see how different philosophers interpreted this text. Modern translators often follow certain commentarial traditions (with or without saying so explicitly).

13.3 About the Reading

This portion of the *Bhagavadgītā* seems to describe an ongoing sequence—indeed, the next verse, 16, talks about a "wheel" (चक्र, *cakra*) that is turning. As Larson (1981, 538) says in his discussion of several translations,

13. Easwaran (2007, 105).

this is a difficult passage, with a range of interpretations going back to early commentators. The problem is what this wheel is. Śaṅkara thinks it describes a cycle involving how Brahman—that most fundamental reality, represented by the syllable (अक्षर, *akṣara*) *oṃ*—brings about the Veda, which commands ritual actions, which results in effects like rain, which brings about food, and which results in people who are themselves Brahman. And these people themselves study the Veda and perform ritual actions, so the wheel continues in a cycle. Rāmānuja, a later commentator, thinks that the अक्षर (*akṣara*) is the imperishable self, which suggests that the wheel turning is the individual embodied self's actions. Famously, Rāmānuja and Śaṅkara disagree about the relationship between self and Brahman, and their competing interpretations demonstrate this.

By their choices, translators can align themselves with competing readings or highlight ambiguities in the original Sanskrit. No single word in English can translate the full set of meanings that are associated with अक्षर (*akṣara*). But the fact that these meanings are all possible makes understanding the text challenging and a rich experience. In the context of the *Bhagavadgītā*, the difference between Śaṅkara and Rāmānuja's analysis is not slight: it is the point of the text that Arjuna should act without desire. Just what this kind of action amounts to and how it is related to reality and Vedic ritual is a central interpretive question.

13.4 Further Resources

If you want to find Sanskrit texts online, you might start at the Indology website:

> Resources for Indological Scholarship. n.d. "External Resources." March 2023. https://indology.info/external-resources/.

There is no single, comprehensive collection of Sanskrit texts online, but the Indology website lists where you can find scans of manuscripts and searchable e-texts in transliteration and Devanāgarī (as well as other

Indic scripts). GRETIL and SARIT are two of the more comprehensive databases listed there, but many others exist. If you work with e-texts, though, be careful since typos can creep in. It's always a good idea to double check with the printed edition the e-text is based on, at minimum.

Learning about critical editions and textual scholarship is not easy for a beginner. As far as I know, no introductory book for Sanskrit text-critical methods is available. Most resources are for biblical literature or ancient Greek and Latin texts. There is an open-access introduction to comparative manuscript studies in what's often called "Oriental Studies," though it does not include Sanskrit:

> Universität Hamburg. 2023. "Comparative Oriental Manuscript Studies: An Introduction." https://www.aai.uni-hamburg.de/en/comst/publications/handbook.html.

The field of translation studies is vast, and the history of the European (and American) study of Sanskrit, now known as "Indology," is likewise complex and wide. A collection of papers on the relationship between the "West" and broadly Hindu Sanskrit literature is one place to dip into long-standing conversations on translation, meaning, philology, and more:

> Sherma, Rita D., and Arvind Sharma, eds. 2008. *Hermeneutics and Hindu Thought: Toward a Fusion of Horizons*. Dordrecht: Springer Science+Business Media B.V.

A similarly themed edited volume collects essays on translation studies for Buddhist texts (not all of which are written in Sanskrit):

> Collett, Alice, ed. 2021. *Translating Buddhism: Historical and Contextual Perspectives*. Albany: State University of New York Press.

Self-Quiz Answer

$\acute{S}_1$ and the other variants include *yajñaḥ* as part of the compound, which is what the hyphen indicates.

यज्ञाद्भवति पर्जन्यो **यज्ञ**कर्मसमुद्भवः
yajñād bhavati parjanyo **yajña**karmasamudbhavaḥ

Afterword: Google Translate for Sanskrit

While I was writing this book, Google announced that it had added Sanskrit to the languages available on its free machine translation platform, available at translate.google.com.[1] Doesn't this technology make my book obsolete, to be thrown into a pile with other outdated books like *Netscape for Dummies* and *How to Use Your Eight-Track Player*? Not quite. In fact, I think the availability of translating tools like Google makes this book even more important. That's because artificial intelligence (AI) translations give us the illusion of perfect accuracy and instant gratification, although the results can have subtle—and sometimes obvious!—errors. Unless you have some understanding of the language you're translating from (the source language) and the one you're translating to (the target language), it would be easy to pop some Sanskrit into Google Translate and mistake the results as authoritative. Below are just two examples. Google may resolve these specific cases by the time you try them out since translation software online is constantly adapting. But the principle they illustrate remains the same: user, beware!

Depending on how you enter the text into Google Translate, the algorithm will give you different results. (Note: it will only accept Sanskrit in Devanāgarī as of this book's writing, not transliterated IAST or other scripts.) The results will differ if you enter a string of text with final punctuation or without. What follows is the same passage, taken from Lesson 8. I have entered it with different punctuation (with and without the *daṇḍas* dividing the verse), and below each passage, I include the results from Google Translate.

1. For the announcement, see Casswell (2022); for the technical details, see Caswell and Bapna, (2022).

A.

यस्य मित्रेण सम्भाषो यस्य मित्रेण संस्थितिः ।
यस्य मित्रेण संलापस्ततो नास्तीह पुण्यवान् ॥

conversation with a friend is a relationship with a friend
There is no pious man in this world who has a conversation with a friend.

B.

यस्य मित्रेण सम्भाषो यस्य मित्रेण संस्थितिः यस्य मित्रेण संलापस्ततो नास्तीह पुण्यवान् ॥

There is no pious person in this world who has a conversation with a friend who is present with a friend who has a conversation with a friend.[2]

Translation (A) is incorrect because it does not recognize that the two lines are syntactically related. But through this book, you've learned how to read verses, recognizing that the single and double *daṇḍa* play different roles. Beyond this mistake, the AI does not recognize that the relative pronoun *yasya* is the logical subject of the verse. The AI also takes the nominative nouns, *saṃbhāsaḥ* and *saṃsthitiḥ*, as being in apposition in a nominal sentence. Finally, it inverts the meaning of the verse in its translation of the last sentence. While it correctly understands *nāsti* as "there is not," it fails to appreciate the ablative *tataḥ* as referring to the person picked out by *yasya* and as the one compared to the pious person. Simply by removing the punctuation, (B) fixes many of these issues. The AI now appreciates the relative-correlative construction. But it still does not recognize that the ablative *tataḥ* means "beyond that one" or "more than that one." Thus, the translation entirely obscures the meaning of the verse. Instead of the most auspicious or happiest person being the one who has conversations with

2. Translations from Google Translate, generated May 18, 2022, https://translate.google.com/.

a friend, someone who has conversations with a friend is *not* auspicious or happy (rendered here as "pious").

Maybe I'm being too hard on Google, giving it something as advanced as Lesson 8. (A note: as a beginning Sanskrit student, I was given the *Hitopadeśa* to read—this is considered an elementary text.) And it's true: the AI can translate *ahaṃ brahmāsmi* correctly, which is the sentence from Lesson 4. So, let's check how it does with Lesson 2 and our first Sanskrit sentence. Here we'll see another issue to be cautious about: word choice in translation.

Lesson 2: Word Choice

A.

योगश्चित्तवृत्तिनिरोधः

Yoga is the restraint of mindfulness

B.

योगश्चित्तवृत्तिनिरोधः ।

Yoga is the restraint of the mind's instincts.

C.

योगश्चित्तवृत्तिनिरोधः.

Yoga is the inhibition of mindfulness.[3]

Again, depending on punctuation, the AI translates the sentence differently. However, none of these are very good, and some are wrong. One problem with (A) and (C) is that "mindfulness" in modern English refers to a kind of meditation. But as we saw, *cittavṛtti* is a broader

3. Translations from Google Translate, generated on May 18, 2022, https://translate.google.com/.

term—it's mental activities in general. In this way, (B) is a bit better, but it's unclear what "mind's instincts" refers to. Are these habits of mind? If so, again, this is too narrow.

The Larger Problem

Aside from the grammatical and lexical issues, there's a larger problem looming over the Google Translate Sanskrit project. That's the question of what it's for. Typically, machine translation isn't intended for literary or philosophical texts. Instead, it's for "everyday life," as one introduction puts it.[4] If that's right, then which Sanskrit texts will we use Google Translate for? While there is an interest in what's called "Spoken Sanskrit," especially in India and (usually) among Hindu members of the Indian diaspora, this version of Sanskrit is not Classical or Vedic Sanskrit. It often draws on contemporary Indian languages, it creates vocabulary for modern things like the Internet and cars using imaginative compounds, and it's typically simple in its syntax.[5] Being able to produce and read these kinds of Sanskrit sentences is indeed a feat of translation technology! However, this does not mean the AI is able to help modern readers understand the vast literature written in Sanskrit.[6]

The texts we've looked at in this book are not "everyday" in the sense of ordinary modern publications. They include philosophy, poetry, literature, and more. All of them are premodern. This makes machine

4. See Poibeau (2017, 4). Book-length introductions to machine translation get outdated quickly, but this one is relatively recent.

5. See Deshpande (2011) for a discussion that situates modern vernacular efforts into the history of the Sanskrit language and Hastings (2003) for a focused analysis of the simplification involved in modern spoken Sanskrit organizations.

6. I have not looked at Sanskrit to Hindi, to German, to French, or any of the other many languages available using the Google Translate platform. I anticipate each would have their own quirks. Anyway, the point of this discussion is not to evaluate the AI, but to explain why it's important to be cautious in using such a tool.

translation of these texts a significant challenge. And Sanskrit vocabulary and even syntax vary according to genre, as well as time period and author—something you will learn as you advance in your study of the language.

Please understand that I'm not saying that Google Translate and other AI translation projects aren't worthwhile or that they will never be able to translate as accurately as human beings do. We don't know the limitations of AI, and how human beings understand language is a question still being investigated. That said, just from how machine translation handles the sample sentences in this overview book, we can see that there is still no replacement for human linguistic abilities. So, use online translation tools as you explore Sanskrit, but do so with other Sanskrit tools at your side—a trusty grammar and dictionary or two!

Appendix 1: Tables

The following tables are a useful reference for the examples in this overview. They are by no means comprehensive. You can find complete tables online and in grammar books (see the references at the end of the Introduction).

Sanskrit Writing and Sound System

Vowels

Vowels in gray are very infrequently encountered, so we do not learn them in this book. They're included below to help you navigate a Sanskrit dictionary.

Vowels

Short Vowel	Long Vowel
अ a - but	आ ā - bawdy
इ i - bit	ई ī - bee
उ u - put	ऊ ū - pool
ऋ ṛ - rig	ॠ ṝ - rig
ऌ ḷ - able	ॡ ḹ - able
ए e - bait	ऐ ai - bite
ओ o - rote	औ au - round

Consonants

The consonants are presented in order of their points of articulation in the mouth. Thick lines around sections of the table indicate which groups are ordered together in dictionaries (see next section).

Consonants

Point of Articulation	Consonants					Semi-Vowels	Sibilants	ह
Voice/aspir	-V / - A	-V / + A	+V / - A	+V / + A	+V / - A	+V / - A	- V / + A	+V / + A
Guttural	क ka	ख kha	ग ga	घ gha	ङ ṅa			ह ha
Palatal	च ca	छ cha	ज ja	झ jha	ञ ña	य ya	श śa	
Retroflex	ट ṭa	ठ ṭha	ड ḍa	ढ ḍha	ण ṇa	र ra	ष ṣa	
Dental	त ta	थ tha	द da	ध dha	न na	ल la	स sa	
Labial	प pa	फ pha	ब ba	भ bha	म ma	व va		

Sanskrit "Alphabet" Order for Dictionaries

Vowels come first, then the consonants in the order of each row (guttural, palatal, etc.) up to the nasals (*na . . . ma*). Then the semi-vowels (*ya . . . va*) and finally the sibilants (*śa . . . sa*), ending with *ha*. The *anusvāra* (*ṃ*) makes things complicated, as sometimes the *ṃ* is used to represent nasals rather than the "true" *anusvāra*. Check the introduction of the dictionary you're using for notation and order.

अ a आ ā इ i ई ī उ u ऊ ū ऋ ṛ ॠ ṝ ऌ ḷ ॡ ḹ ए e ऐ ai ओ o औ au
अं aṃ
क ka ख kha ग ga घ gha ङ ṅa
च ca छ cha ज ja झ jha ञ ña
ट ṭa ठ ṭha ड ḍa ढ ḍha ण ṇa

त ta थ tha द da ध dha न na
प pa फ pha ब ba भ bha म ma
य ya र ra ल la व va श śa ष ṣa स sa ह ha

Numerals

Numerals in Devanāgarī are below. (For numbers—that is, words like "one," "two," and so on—consult a dictionary or grammar.)

Numerals

Devanāgarī	Transliteration
१	1
२	2
३	3
४	4
५	5
६	6
७	7
८	8
९	9
०	0

Declensions

a-stem, masculine, योग (*yoga*)

	Singular	Dual	Plural
Nominative	योगः	योगौ	योगाः
Accusative	योगम्	योगौ	योगान्
Instrumental	योगेन	योगाभ्याम्	योगैः
Dative	योगाय	योगाभ्याम्	योगेभ्यः
Ablative	योगात्	योगाभ्याम्	योगेभ्यः
Genitive	योगस्य	योगयोः	योगानाम्
Locative	योगे	योगयोः	योगेषु
Vocative	योग	योगौ	योगाः

a-stem, neuter, वन (*vana*)

	Singular	Dual	Plural
Nominative	वनम्	वने	वनानि
Accusative	वनम्	वने	वनानि
Instrumental	वनेन	वनाभ्याम्	वनैः
Dative	वनाय	वनाभ्याम्	वनेभ्यः
Ablative	वनात्	वनाभ्याम्	वनेभ्यः
Genitive	वनस्य	वनयोः	वनानाम्
Locative	वने	वनयोः	वनेषु
Vocative	वन	वने	वनानि

ā-stem, feminine, कन्या (*kanyā*)

	Singular	Dual	Plural
Nominative	कन्या	कन्ये	कन्याः
Accusative	कन्याम्	कन्ये	कन्याः
Instrumental	कन्यया	कन्याभ्याम्	कन्याभिः
Dative	कन्यायै	कन्याभ्याम्	कन्याभ्यः
Ablative	कन्यायाः	कन्याभ्याम्	कन्याभ्यः
Genitive	कन्यायाः	कन्ययोः	कन्यानाम्
Locative	कन्यायाम्	कन्ययोः	कन्यासु
Vocative	कन्ये	कन्ये	कन्याः

an-stem, masculine, आत्मन् (*ātman*)

	Singular	Dual	Plural
Nominative	आत्मा	आत्मानौ	आत्मानः
Accusative	आत्मानम्	आत्मानौ	आत्मनः
Instrumental	आत्मना	आत्मभ्याम्	आत्मभिः
Dative	आत्मने	आत्मभ्याम्	आत्मभ्यः
Ablative	आत्मनः	आत्मभ्याम्	आत्मभ्यः
Genitive	आत्मनः	आत्मनोः	आत्मनाम्
Locative	आत्मनि	आत्मनोः	आत्मसु
Vocative	आत्मन्	आत्मानौ	आत्मानः

an-stem, neuter, कर्मन् (*karman*)

	Singular	Dual	Plural
Nominative	कर्म	कर्मणी	कर्माणि
Accusative	कर्म	कर्मणी	कर्माणि
Instrumental	कर्मणा	कर्मभ्याम्	कर्मभिः
Dative	कर्मणे	कर्मभ्याम्	कर्मभ्यः
Ablative	कर्मणः	कर्मभ्याम्	कर्मभ्यः
Genitive	कर्मणः	कर्मणोः	कर्मणाम्
Locative	कर्मणि	कर्मणोः	कर्मसु
Vocative	कर्म / कर्मन्	कर्मणी	कर्माणि

i-stem, feminine, प्रकृति (*prakṛti*)

	Singular	Dual	Plural
Nominative	प्रकृतिः	प्रकृती	प्रकृतयः
Accusative	प्रकृतिम्	प्रकृती	प्रकृतीः
Instrumental	प्रकृत्या	प्रकृतिभ्याम्	प्रकृतिभिः
Dative	प्रकृत्यै / प्रकृतये	प्रकृतिभ्याम्	प्रकृतिभ्यः
Ablative	प्रकृत्याः / प्रकृतेः	प्रकृतिभ्याम्	प्रकृतिभ्यः
Genitive	प्रकृत्याः / प्रकृतेः	प्रकृत्योः	प्रकृतीनाम्
Locative	प्रकृत्याम् / प्रकृतौ	प्रकृत्योः	प्रकृतिषु
Vocative	प्रकृते	प्रकृती	प्रकृतयः

first-person pronoun, अस्मद् (*asmad*)

Optional shortened forms (enclitics) after the forward slash

	Singular	Dual	Plural
Nominative	अहम्	आवाम्	वयम्
Accusative	माम् / मा	आवाम् / नौ	अस्मान् / नः
Instrumental	मया	आवाभ्याम्	अस्माभिः
Dative	मह्यम् / मे	आवाभ्याम् / नौ	अस्मभ्यम् / नः
Ablative	मत्	आवाभ्याम्	अस्मत्
Genitive	मम / मे	आवयोः / नौ	अस्माकम् / नः
Locative	मयि	आवयोः	अस्मासु

second-person pronoun, युष्मद् (*yuṣmad*)

Optional shortened forms (enclitics) after the forward slash

	Singular	Dual	Plural
Nominative	त्वम्	युवाम्	यूयम्
Accusative	त्वाम् / त्वा	युवाम् / वाम्	युष्मान् / वः
Instrumental	त्वया	युवाभ्याम्	युष्माभिः
Dative	तुभ्यम् / ते	युवाभ्याम् / वाम्	युष्मभ्यम् / वः
Ablative	त्वत्	युवाभ्याम्	युष्मत्
Genitive	तव / ते	युवयोः / वाम्	युष्माकम् / वः
Locative	त्वयि	युवयोः	युष्मासु

demonstrative pronoun, neuter, तद् (*tad*)

	Singular	Dual	Plural
Nominative	तत्	ते	तानि
Accusative	तत्	ते	तानि
Instrumental	तेन	ताभ्याम्	तैः
Dative	तस्मै	ताभ्याम्	तेभ्यः
Ablative	तस्मात्	ताभ्याम्	तेभ्यः
Genitive	तस्य	तयोः	तेषाम्
Locative	तस्मिन्	तयोः	तेषु

demonstrative pronoun, neuter, इदम् (*idam*)

	Singular	Dual	Plural
Nominative	इदम्	इमे	इमानि
Accusative	इदम्	इमे	इमानि
Instrumental	तेन	ताभ्याम्	तैः
Dative	तस्मै	ताभ्याम्	तेभ्यः
Ablative	तस्मात्	ताभ्याम्	तेभ्यः
Genitive	तस्य	तयोः	तेषाम्
Locative	तस्मिन्	तयोः	तेषु

demonstrative pronoun, neuter, एतद् (*etad*)

	Singular	Dual	Plural
Nominative	एतत्	एते	एतानि
Accusative	एतत्	एते	एतानि
Instrumental	एतेन	एताभ्याम्	एतैः
Dative	एतस्मै	एताभ्याम्	एतेभ्यः
Ablative	एतस्मात्	एताभ्याम्	एतेभ्यः
Genitive	एतस्य	एतयोः	एतेषाम्
Locative	एतस्मिन्	एतयोः	एतेषु

relative pronoun, masculine, यद् (*yad*)

	Singular	Dual	Plural
Nominative	यः	यौ	ये
Accusative	यम्	यौ	यान्
Instrumental	येन	याभ्याम्	यैः
Dative	यस्मै	याभ्याम्	येभ्यः
Ablative	यस्मात्	याभ्याम्	येभ्यः
Genitive	यस्य	ययोः	येषाम्
Locative	यस्मिन्	ययोः	येषु

Verb Conjugations

present indicative √भू (*bhū*) (1P) - to be, to exist

	Singular	Dual	Plural
Third person	भवति (bhava**ti**) - he/she/it is	भवतः (bhava**taḥ**) - those two are	भवन्ति (bhava**nti**) - they are
Second person	भवसि (bhava**si**) - you are	भवथः (bhava**thaḥ**) - you two are	भवथ (bhava**tha**) - you all are
First person	भवामि (bhav**āmi**) - I am	भवावः (bhav**āvaḥ**) - we two are	भवामः (bhav**āmaḥ**) - we are

present indicative √भू (*bhū*) (1A) - to be, to exist

	Singular	Dual	Plural
Third person	भवते (bhava**te**) - he/she/it is	भवेते (bhav**ete**) - those two are	भवन्ते (bhava**nte**) - they are
Second person	भवसे (bhava**se**) - you are	भवेथे (bhav**ethe**) - you two are	भवध्वे (bhava**dhve**) - you all are
First person	भवे (bhav**e**) - I am	भवावहे (bhav**āvahe**) - we two are	भवामहे (bhav**āmahe**) - we are

present optative √भू (*bhū*) (1P) - to be, to exist

	Singular	Dual	Plural
Third person	भवेत् (bhav**et**) - he/she/could be	भवेताम् (bhav**etām**) - those two could be	भवेयुः (bhav**eyuḥ**) – could be
Second person	भवेः (bhav**eḥ**) - you could be	भवेतम् (bhav**etam**) - you two could be	भवेत (bhav**eta**) - you could be
First person	भवेयम् (bhav**eyam**) - I could be	भवेव (bhav**eva**) – we two could be	भवेम (bhav**ema**) - we could be

present indicative √अस् (*as*) (2P) - to be, to exist

	Singular	**Dual**	**Plural**
	Strong stem	***Weak stem***	
Third person	अस्ति (as**ti**) - he/she/it is	स्तः (s**taḥ**) - those two are	सन्ति (s**anti**) - they are
Second person	असि (a**si**) - you are	स्थः (s**thaḥ**) - you two are	स्थ (st**ha**) - you all are
First person	अस्मि (as**mi**) - I am	स्वः (s**vaḥ**) - we two are	स्मः (s**maḥ**) - we are

present indicative √कृ (*kṛ*) (8P) - to make, to do, to cause

	Singular	**Dual**	**Plural**
	Strong stem	***Weak stem***	
Third person	करोति (karo**ti**) - he/she/it makes	कुरुतः (kuru**taḥ**) - those two make	कुर्वन्ति (kurv**anti**) - they make
Second person	करोषि (karo**ṣi**) - you make	कुरुथः (kuru**thaḥ**) - you two make	कुरुथ (kuru**tha**) - you all make
First person	करोमि (karo**mi**) - I make	कुर्वः (kur**vaḥ**) - we two make	कुर्मः (kur**maḥ**) - we make

Appendix 2: Sanskrit Glossary

Devanāgarī	Transliteration	Gender/Part of Speech	Translation	Lesson
ं	ṃ (the *anusvāra*)	a symbol for nasal consonant		4
।, ॥	.	punctuation mark (*daṇḍa*) which singly acts as a period; doubly acts as a full stop at the end of a verse or section		2
१	1	num.	one (other numerals are in Appendix 1)	2
अक्ष	akṣa	neut. n.	sense faculty	11
अक्षर	akṣara	neut. n.	lit., imperishable (*a-kṣara*); sound, syllable; the syllable *om* (ॐ)	4, 13
अग्नौ	agnau	masc. loc. sg. n.	about fire; in fire	3
अनुमान	anumāna	neut. n.	an inference	3, 11
अन्तःकरण	antaḥkaraṇa	neut. n.	internal faculty (like the mind)	11
अन्न	anna	neut. n.	food; rice	13
अन्यस्मिन्	anyasmin	masc. loc. sg. adj.	in another, in something else	10
अभाव	abhāva	masc. n.	absence, lack, (lit., nonbeing)	10

Devanāgarī	Transliteration	Gender/Part of Speech	Translation	Lesson
अभिधर्म	abhidharma	masc. n.	Buddhist teachings about metaphysics	10
अभिधान	abhidhāna	neut. n.	designation, term, word	10
अभिधेय	abhidheya	gerundive (future ps. ptp.)	referent, object of a word (lit., what is to be designated)	10
अभिप्राय	abhiprāya	masc. n.	thought, idea	11
अर्थशास्त्र	arthaśāstra	masc. n., cpd.	*Treatise on Success* (title)	7
अश्व	aśva	masc. n.	horse	3
√अस्	√as	v. (2P)	to be, to exist (see section 3.2.3 to understand the √ symbol)	4
अस्मद्	asmad	1 pn.	I/we	4, 6
आक्षिपति	ākṣipati	pres. indc. 3 sg. from ā + √*kṣip* (6P)	he/she/ one replies, responds	11
आत्मन्	ātman	masc. n.	self	10
√आप् (+प्र)	√āp (+ pra)	v. (5P)	attained, acquired, reached	9
आरण्यक	āraṇyaka	neut. n.	name for a type of text recited in a forest	4
आसन	āsana	neut. n.	posture, pose	2
आह	āha	v., perfect 3 sg. from √*āh* (reconstructed form)	he/she/one says	11

Devanāgarī	Transliteration	Gender/Part of Speech	Translation	Lesson
इति	iti	indc.	"" (quotation marker)	5
इदम्	idam	neut. pn.	this	6
इव	iva	indc.	like, as if	9
इह	iha	indc.	now, here	8
उत्तम	uttama	adj.	highest; best	9
उद्	ud	pfx.	out of, from	13
उपकार	upakāra	masc. n.	assistance, help	7
उपदेश	upadeśa	masc. n.	instruction	8
उपनिषद्	upaniṣad	fem. n.	name for texts that contain teachings about the self, existence, ritual	4
उपमान	upamāna	neut. n.	comparison, analogy	11
एतद्	etad	neut. pn.	this	6
एव	eva	ind.	indeed, really, truly	9
कण्ठ	kaṇṭha	masc. n.	throat, neck	11
कथम्	katham	intr.	how (question)	10
कन्या	kanyā	fem. noun	girl, young woman	9, 11
कर्मन्	karman	neut. n.	action, activity, effort	5
काम	kāma	masc. n.	desire, love	5
काव्य	kāvya	neut. n.	poetry	12
कीकस	kīkasa	neut. n.	bone	11

Devanāgarī	Transliteration	Gender/Part of Speech	Translation	Lesson
कोश	kośa	masc. n.	treasury, storehouse	10
√कृ (+ उप)	√*kṛ* (+ upa)	v. (8P)	assist, help	7
गच्छति	gacchati	v. (1P), 3 sg. v. from √*gam*	he/she/it travels, goes	3
√गम्	√*gam*	v. (1P)	understands; goes (Lesson 3)	10
ग्राम	grāma	masc. n.	village, town	3
च	ca	indc.	and	2
चन्द्र	candra	masc. n.	moon	12
चित्त	citta	neut. n.	thought, awareness	2
चेत्	cet	indc.	could be, might be (with *iti*)	11
जगत्	jagat	neut. n.	universe, world	12
जरा	jarā	fem. n.	old age	9
टीका	ṭīkā	fem. nm. sg. n.	gloss, notes (kind of commentary)	2
ततः	tataḥ	indc.	thus, therefore	8
तत्	tat	neut. nm. sg. pn.	it, that	2
तद्	tad	neut. pn. (stem form)	that	6
तथागत	tathāgata	masc. n.	the one who has gone/ come in such a way	10
तात्पर्य	tātparya	neut. n.	intention, aim	11

Devanāgarī	Transliteration	Gender/Part of Speech	Translation	Lesson
तावत्	tāvat	correlative pn.	to the extent that	7, 8
तृतीया	tṛtīyā	fem. n.	third	8
ते	te	2 pn. d.	for you, to you	2
दम्य	damya	gdv.	able to be trained, tamed	2
दर्शन	darśana	neut. n.	experience, observation	3
देव	deva	masc. n.	god, deity	2
धर्म	dharma	masc. n.	righteousness, religion, ethical principle, law, rule	3
धूम	dhūma	masc. n.	smoke	3
न	na	ind.	no (negation of verb)	5
ननु	nanu	indc.	discourse marker indicating objection in what follows: "But couldn't it be that?," "is it not that"	11
नमः	namaḥ	neut. nom. sg. n.	honor	2
नित्य	nitya	adj.	eternal, permanent	9, 13
निरोध	nirodha	masc. n.	stopping, cessation, restraint	2
निर्वर्त्तन	nirvarttana	neut. n.	accomplishing, completing	11

Devanāgarī	Transliteration	Gender/Part of Speech	Translation	Lesson
निर्वाण	nirvāṇa	neut. n.	blowing out, extinction	5
निष्-	niṣ-	pfx.	without, non-	5
नीति	nīti	fem. n.	leadership; good conduct	7
नील	nīla	adj.	dark color, dark blue	11
न्याय	nyāya	masc. n.	right reason, rule; name of philosophical tradition	3
पद	pada	masc. n.	word	12
पदच्छेद	padaccheda	masc. n.	word-division	11
पद्म	padma	neut. n.	lotus	9
परमेश्वर	parameśvara	masc. n., cpd. (*parama* + *īśvara*)	highest lord (Śiva)	12
पर्जन्य	parjanya	masc. n. (or proper name)	rain; Parjanya god of rain	13
√पश्	√paś	v. (4P)	sees, views	10
पार्वती	pārvatī	fem. n., proper name	Pārvatī (Śiva's wife)	12
पिता	pitā	masc. sg. nom. n.	father	12
पुण्यवान्	puṇyavān	adj., masc. nom. sg.	one who is pious, righteous	8
पुत्र	putra	masc. n.	son	11
पुनर्	punar	indc.	then (with *katham*)	10
पुरुष	puruṣa	masc. n.	person, man	2
पुस्तक	pustaka	neut. n.	book	2

Devanāgarī	Transliteration	Gender/Part of Speech	Translation	Lesson
पूर्वपक्ष	pūrvapakṣa	masc. n., cpd.	earlier position (in a debate, the opponent view)	7
प्रकृति	prakṛti	fem. n.	form, pattern	8
प्रज्ञा	prajñā	fem. n.	knowledge, wisdom	11
प्रति	prati	pfx.	toward, for; for each	11
प्रतिपत्ति	pratipatti	fem. n.	understanding, knowing, acquiring	12
प्रतिष्ठिता	pratiṣṭhitā	fem. nom. sg. ppp. (as adj. from प्रति + √स्था, 1P)	being in a fixed, firm state	11
प्रत्यक्ष	pratyakṣa	neut. n.	perception	3, 11
प्रधान	pradhāna	neut. n.	predominant thing; origin	8
प्रमाण	pramāṇa	neut. n.	way of knowing, knowledge source	11
प्रयोजन	prayojana	neut n.	purpose, goal	5
प्राप्त	prāpta	ppp.	has been acquired	9
बहु	bahu	adj.	many, much, a lot	5
बुद्ध	buddha	masc. n.	the Buddha (lit., "enlightened one" or "awakened one")	3
√बुध्	√budh	v. (1P)	understand, learn	7

Devanāgarī	Transliteration	Gender/Part of Speech	Translation	Lesson
बृहत्	bṛhat	adj.	great	4
ब्रह्म	brahma	n., neut. nom. sg. form of *brahman*	the Absolute, the divine; truth; the Vedas	4
भद्र	bhadra	neut. n.	prosperity, good fortune	5
भव (+ सम्, + उद्)	bhava (+ sam, + ud)	masc. n.	coming into existence, production, origin.	13
भारत	bhārata	masc. n.	descendants of Bharata	9
भावः	bhāva	masc. n.	meaning, idea (esp. with *iti*)	11
√भू	√bhū	v. (1P)	to be, to exist	3, 7
भूत	bhūta	adj. (ppp. from √*bhū*, (1P)	lit., what has become; being	13
महत्	mahat	adj.	great	9
महा-	mahā-	adj., cpd. form of *mahat*	great, noble	2
माता	mātā	fem. sg. nom. n.	mother	12
मित्र	mitra	neut. n.	friend, ally	7, 8
मुख	mukha	neut. n.	face, mouth	9, 11, 12
यज्ञ	yajña	masc. n.	offering, sacrifice; worship, devotion	13
यदि	yadi	indc.	if	10
यावत्	yāvat	rel. pn.	to the extent that	7
युष्मद्	yuṣmad	2 pn.	you	6

Devanāgarī	Transliteration	Gender/Part of Speech	Translation	Lesson
योग	yoga	masc. n.	discipline, method, practice	1, 2
रघुवंश	raghuvaṃśa	masc. n., cpd. (*raghu* + *vaṃśa*)	lineage of Raghu	12
राजा	rājā	masc. nom. sg. n.	king, leader	2
√राज्	√rāj	v. (1P)	rule, govern	9
राज्य	rājya	neut. n.	kingdom	3, 9
राम	rāma	masc. n., proper name	Rāma	3
रूप	rūpa	neut. n.	beauty; physical form	9
लक्षण	lakṣaṇa	neut. n.	characteristic, definition	7
लोक	loka	masc. n.	world, ordinary people	12
वन	vana	neut. n.	forest	3
वन्दे	vande	1 pres. ind. sg. (√*vand*, 1A)	I praise, I honor, I adore, etc.	12
वाक्य	vākya	neut. n.	sentence	4
वाक्ष्यमाणाः	vakṣyamāṇāḥ	future ptp., fem. nom. pl. from √*vac* (2P)	what will be said later, what needs to be mentioned	11
वाच् (वाग्)	vāc (vāg)	fem. n. (-*g* with sandhi)	speech, language	12
वात्स्यायन	vātsyāyana	masc. n., proper name	Vātsyāyana	5

Devanāgarī	Transliteration	Gender/Part of Speech	Translation	Lesson
विग्रह	vigraha	masc. n.	analysis (of compound), separation into its parts	11
विद्धि	viddhi	2 sg., impv. from √*vid* (2P)	you, know!	13
विनय	vinaya	masc. n.	discipline, restraint	9
विन्दसि	vindasi	2 sg., pres. indc. v. from √*vid* (6P)	you think (second person present indicative)	7
विषय	viṣaya	masc. n.	object, content of an experience	11
√वृत्	√vṛt	v. (1A)	engaged in, done, employed; applies to (with locative case), in the sense of a word being used for something	9, 10
वृत्ति	vṛtti	fem. n.	movement, activity	2
व्रीहि	vrīhi	masc. n.	rice	5
शब्द	śabda	masc. n.	speech, language, testimony	11, 12
शिष्य	śiṣya	masc. n.	student	2
शेष	śeṣa	masc. n.	remainder, what must be supplied (with *iti*)	11

Devanāgarī	Transliteration	Gender/Part of Speech	Translation	Lesson
शोक	śoka	masc. n.	grief, sorrow	8
श्री	śrī	fem. n.	name of Lakṣmī; prosperity, wealth, success	9
श्लोक	śloka	masc. n.	name of a meter; sound, call	8
श्वेतकेतु	śvetaketu	masc. proper name	Śvetaketu	6
संपृक्त	saṃpṛkta	ppp. (*sam* + √*pṛc*, 7P)	intermixed, inseparable	12
संबद्ध	saṃbaddha	ppp. (*sam* + √*badh*, 10P)	tightly connected, related, a relationship	12
संलाप	saṃlāpa	masc. n.	conversation, chatter	8
संस्थिति	saṃsthiti	fem. n.	union, connection	8
सम्भाष	sambhāṣa	masc. n.	conversation, discourse	8
सर्व	sarva	adj.	all, every	13
सागर	sāgara	masc. n.	ocean	3
सांप्रतम्	sāṃpratam	indc. (adv.)	appropriately, suitably	9
सारथि	sārathi	masc. n.	charioteer	2
सुव्यक्तम्	suvyaktam	adv.	clearly, distinctly	10
सूत्र	sūtra	neut. n.	short saying, aphorism; thread	2
स्कन्ध	skandha	masc. n.	heap, aggregate	10

Devanāgarī	Transliteration	Gender/Part of Speech	Translation	Lesson
स्थित	sthita	ppp. (as adj. from √*sthā*, 1P)	being in a particular state	11
√हन्	√han	v. (2P)	destroy, kill	9
हन्ति	hanti	3 sg. √*han* (2P)	he/she/it destroys	9
हि	hi	indc.	for, because	9
हित	hita	neut. n.	what is appropriate, useful, beneficial	8
हितोपदेश	hitopadeśa	masc. n., cpd.	*Instruction in What is Appropriate* (title)	8
हे	he	ptc.	Hey!; oh! (direct address)	6

Bibliography

Ajotikar, Tanuja P, and Malhar Kulkarni. 2016. "Adverbs in the Sanskrit Wordnet." In *GWC 2016 Proceedings of the 8th Global Wordnet Conference*, edited by Verginica Mititelu, Corina Forăscu, Christiane Fellbaum, and Piek Vossen, 8. Bucharest, Romania: Global Wordnet Association.

Ali, Daud. 2004. *Courtly Culture and Political Life in Early Medieval India*. Cambridge: Cambridge University Press.

Apte, V. S. 1925. *The Student's Guide to Sanskrit Composition*. 9th ed. Bombay: The Standard Publishing Company.

Balogh, Dániel, and Arlo Griffiths. 2020. "DHARMA Transliteration Guide." https://hal.science/halshs-02272407.

Belvalkar, Shripad Krishna, ed. 1968. *The Bhagavadgītā: Being Reprint of Relevant Parts of Bhīṣmaparvan from B.O.R. Institute's Edition of the Mahābhārata*. Pune: Bhandarkar Oriental Research Institute.

Brereton, Joel. 1986. "'Tat Tvam Asi' in Context." *Zeitschrift Der Deutschen Morgenlandischen Gesellschaft* 136 (1): 98–109.

Bronner, Yigal. 2007. "This Is No Lotus, It Is a Face: Poetics as Grammar in Daṇḍin's Investigation." In *The Poetics of Grammar and the Metaphysics of Sound*, edited by Sergio La Porta and David Shulman. Jerusalem: Jerusalem Studies in Religion and Culture, 6. Brill.

———. 2010. *Extreme Poetry: The South Asian Movement of Simultaneous Narration*. New York: Columbia University Press.

Bryant, Edwin F. 2015. *The Yoga Sutras of Patañjali: A New Edition, Translation, and Commentary*. New York: Farrar, Straus and Giroux.

Cardona, George. 1974. "Pāṇini's Kārakās: Agency, Animation and Identity." *Journal of Indian Philosophy* 2: 231–306.

———. 1988. *Pāṇini: His Work and Its Traditions. Part I: General Introduction and Background*. Delhi: Motilal Banarsidass.

Casswell, Isaac. 2022. "Google Translate Learns 24 New Languages." The Keyword (blog). May 11, 2022. https://blog.google/products/translate/24-new-languages/.

Casswell, Isaac and Ankur Bapna. 2022. "Unlocking Zero-Resource Machine Translation to Support New Languages in Google Translate." Google Research (blog). May 11, 2022. https://ai.googleblog.com/2022/05/24-new-languages-google-translate.html.

Chakrabarti, Arindam. 2016. "'Now, Kālī, I Shall Eat You Up!': On the Logic of the Vocative." In *Ramchandra Gandhi: The Man and His Philosophy*, edited by A. Raghuramaraju, 194–208. New Delhi: Routledge. Dairianathan, Eugene. 2012. "The Burden of Song: Vedic Metal in Singapore." *Journal of Creative Communications* 7 (3): 243–60.

Dasti, Matthew R. 2023. *Vātsyāyana's* Commentary on the Nyāya-sūtra: *A Guide*. Oxford: Oxford University Press.

Dasti, Matthew R., and Stephen H. Phillips. 2017. *The Nyāya-sūtra: Selections with Early Commentaries*. Indianapolis: Hackett Publishing Company, Inc.

Deshpande, Madhav M. 2011. "Efforts to Vernacularize Sanskrit: Degree of Success and Failure." In *Handbook of Language & Ethnic Identity*, edited by Joshua A. Fishman and Ofelia García, 2:218–29. Oxford: Oxford University Press.

Deutsch, Eliot. 1968. *The Bhagavad Gītā*. Lanham, MD: University Press of America.

Doniger, Wendy. 2009. "How to Escape the Curse." Review of *The Mahabharata*, by John Smith. *London Review of Books* (October 8, 2009). https://www.lrb.co.uk/the-paper/v31/n19/wendy-doniger/how-to-escape-the-curse.

———. 2016. *Redeeming the Kamasutra*. Oxford: Oxford University Press.

Downing, Angela. 2015. *English Grammar: A University Course*. 3rd ed. New York: Routledge.

Dundas, Paul, trans. 2017. *Magha: The Killing of Shishupala*. Murty Classical Library of India, 11. Cambridge: Harvard University Press.

Easwaran, Eknath. 2007. *The Bhagavad Gita*. Tomales, CA: Nilgiri Press.

Eltschinger, Vincent. 2017. "Why Did the Buddhists Adopt Sanskrit?" *Open Linguistics* 3, no. 1: 308–26. https://doi.org/10.1515/opli-2017-0015.

Fitzgerald, James L. 2004. "*Mahābhārata*." In *The Hindu World*. Edited by Sushil Mittal and Gene R. Thursby, 52–74. New York: Routledge.

Gerow, Edwin. 1971. *A Glossary of Indian Figures of Speech*. The Hague: Mouton & Co.

Gillon, Brendan S. 1996. "Word Order in Classical Sanskrit." *Indian Linguistics* 57 (1–4): 1–36.

———. 2007. "Pāṇini's Aṣṭādhyāyī and Linguistic Theory." *Journal of Indian Philosophy* 35 (5): 445–68. https://doi.org/10.1007/s10781-007-9027-3.

Gold, Jonathan C. 2022. "Vasubandhu." In *The Stanford Encyclopedia of Philosophy*, edited by Edward N. Zalta and Uri Nodelman. Metaphysics Research Lab, Stanford University. Winter 2022. https://plato.stanford.edu/archives/win2022/entries/vasubandhu/.

Gombrich, Richard. 1979. "'He Cooks Softly': Adverbs in Sanskrit Grammar." *Bulletin of the School of Oriental and African Studies* 42 (2): 244–56. https://doi.org/10.1017/S0041977X0014580X.

Hahn, Michael. 1982. *Ratnākaraśānti's Chandoratnākara*. Nepal Research Centre Miscellaneous Papers, 34. Kathmandu: Nepal Research Centre.

Hastings, Adi. 2003. "Simplifying Sanskrit." *Pragmatics* 13 (4): 499–513. https://doi.org/10.1075/prag.13.4.03has.

Huang, Po-chi. 2009. "The Cult Of Vetāla And Tantric Fantasy." In *Rethinking Ghosts in World Religions*, 123:211–35. Numen Book Series. Leiden: Brill.

Ingalls, Daniel H. H., Jeffrey Moussaieff Masson, and M. V. Patwardhan, trans. 1990. *The Dhvanyāloka of Ānandavardhana with the Locana of Abhinavagupta*. Cambridge, MA: Harvard University Press.

Keating, Malcolm. 2019. "The Philosophy of the *Bhagavad Gītā*: A Contemporary Introduction by Keya Maitra." *Philosophy East and West* 69 (3).

Kramrisch, Stella. 1992. *The Presence of Śiva*. 2nd ed. Princeton, NJ: Princeton University Press.

Kulkarni, Amba, Preeti Shukla, Pavankumar Satuluri, and Devanad Shukl. 2013. "How Free Is 'Free' Word Order in Sanskrit?" In Conference Proceedings for the Seminar on Sanskrit Syntax and Discourse Structures, Paris, France. https://sanskrit.uohyd.ac.in/faculty/amba/PUBLICATIONS/papers/sktsynOffprintAKulkarnietal.pdf.

Larson, Gerald James. 1981. "The Song Celestial: Two Centuries of the 'Bhagavad Gītā' in English." *Philosophy East and West* 31, no. 4 (October): 513–41.

Matilal, Bimal Krishna. 1989. *Moral Dilemmas in the Mahābhārata*. Delhi: Motilal Banarsidass.

McConnachie, James. 2008. *The Book of Love: The Story of the Kamasutra*. New York: Metropolitan Books.

Mehendale, M. A. 2007. "The Critical Edition of the *Mahābhārata*: Its Achievement and Limitations." *Annals of the Bhandarkar Oriental Research Institute* 88: 1–16.

Naik, Bapurao S. 1971. *Typography of Devanāgarī*. 3 vols. Bombay: Directorate of Languages.

Olivelle, Patrick. 2008. *Upaniṣads: A New Translation by Patrick Olivelle*. Oxford: Oxford University Press.

———. 2016. *King, Governance, and Law in Ancient India: Kautilya's Arthaśāstra*. Oxford: Oxford University Press.

Ollett, Andrew. 2017. *Language of the Snakes: Prakrit, Sanskrit, and the Language Order of Premodern India*. Oakland: University of California Press.

Pal, Supriya Banik. 2010. "Some Women Writers and Their Works in Classical Sanskrit Literature: A Reinterpretation." In *Asian Literary Voices: From Marginal to Mainstream*, edited by Philip F. Williams, 149–60. Amsterdam: Amsterdam University Press.

Patel, Deven M. 2014. *Text to Tradition: The Naiṣadhīyacarita and Literary Community in South Asia*. New York: Columbia University Press.

———. 2022. "The Literary Commentary in Sanskrit as Metalinguistic Communication." *Asiatische Studien / Études Asiatiques* 76, no. 3 (October): 623–41. https://doi.org/10.1515/asia-2021-0037.

Patil, Urmila. 2017. "Friend, Enemy, Frenemy: The Hitopadeśa on Making and Breaking Friendship:" *Studies in History* 33 (1), 7–25. https://doi.org/10.1177/0257643016677443.

Patton, Laurie L. 2008. *The Bhagavad Gita*. Penguin Classics. London: Penguin.

Phillips, Stephen H. 2009. *Yoga, Karma, and Rebirth: A Brief History and Philosophy*. New York: Columbia University Press.

Poibeau, Thierry. 2017. *Machine Translation*. Boston, MA: MIT Press.

Pollock, Sheldon. 2015. "What Was Philology in Sanskrit?" In *World Philology*, edited by Sheldon Pollock, Benjamin A. Elman, and Ku-ming Kevin Chang, 114–36. Cambridge, MA: Harvard University Press.

Preisendanz, Karin. 2008. "Text, Commentary, Annotation: Some Reflections on the Philosophical Genre." *Journal of Indian Philosophy* 36 (5): 599–618.

Saxena, Pooja. n.d. "Devanagari Type Anatomy." Typetogether. Accessed November 20, 2022. https://www.type-together.com/devanagari-type-anatomy.

Staal, J. F. 1967. "Word Order in Sanskrit and Universal Grammar." In *Foundations of Language*. Supplementary Series 5. Dordrecht: D. Reidel Publishing Co.

———. 2003. *A Reader on the Sanskrit Grammarians*. Boston, MA: MIT Press.

Stoler-Miller, Barbara. 1986. *The Bhagavad-Gita: Krishna's Counsel in Time of War*. New York: Random House Publishing.

Taber, John A. 1989. "The Theory of the Sentence in Pūrva Mīmāṃsā and Western Philosophy." *Journal of Indian Philosophy* 17 (4): 407–30.

———. 2016. "Mīmāṃsā." In *Routledge Encyclopedia of Philosophy*, 1st ed. London: Routledge. https://doi.org/10.4324/9780415249126-F008-1.

Thapliyal, Uma Prasad. 2021. *Wars and War-Tactics in Ancient India*. London: Routledge.

Tubb, Gary A. 1984. "Heroine as Hero: Pārvatī in the Kumārasaṃbhava and the Pārvatīpariṇaya." Journal of the American Oriental Society 104 (2): 219–36.

Tubb, Gary Alan, and Emery Robert Boose. 2007. *Scholastic Sanskrit: A Handbook for Students*. New York: American Institute of Buddhist Studies.

Sanskrit Sources for Readings

If no additional source is noted below, I have relied only on publicly available electronic versions of readings on the Göttingen Register of Electronic Texts in Indian Languages (GRETIL), https://gretil.sub.uni-goettingen.de/gretil.html.

Lesson 2: *Yogasūtra* 1.2

Lesson 3: *Nyāyabhāṣya* on *Nyāyasūtra* 2.1.32
Thakur, Anantalal, ed. 1997. *Gautamīyanyāyadarśana with Bhāṣya of Vātsyāyana*. Nyāyacaturgranthikā 1. New Delhi: Indian Council of Philosophical Research.

Lesson 4: *Bṛhadāraṇyaka Upaniṣad* 1.4.10

Lesson 5: *Kāmasūtra* 1.2.30

Lesson 6: *Chāndogya Upaniṣad* 6.8.7

Lesson 7: *Arthaśāstra* 7.9.12

Lesson 8: *Hitopadeśa* 1.39

Lesson 9: *Mahābhārata* 5.34.10

Lesson 10: *Abhidharmakośabhāṣya* 9
Śāstri, Swāmī Dwārikadās, ed. 1987. *Abhidharmakośa & Bhāṣya of Ācarya Vasubandhu with Sphutārthā Commentary of Ācarya Yaśomitra*. Bauddha Bharati 5, 6, 7, 9. Varanasi: Bauddha Bharati.

Lesson 11: *Rājamartaṇḍa* 1.2
Mitra, Rājendralāla, ed. 1883. *The Yoga Aphorisms of Patañjali with the Commentary of Bhoja Rājā and an English Translation by Rājendralāla Mitra*. Calcutta: Asiatic Society of Bengal.

Lesson 12: *Raghuvaṃśa* 1.1
Kale, V. M., ed. 1957. *The Raghuvaṃśa Of Kālidāsa*. 5th ed. Delhi: Motilal Banarsidass.

Lesson 13: *Bhagavadgītā* 3.14–15
Belvalkar, Shripad Krishna, ed. 1968. *The Bhagavadgītā: Being Reprint of Relevant Parts of Bhīṣmaparvan from B.O.R. Institute's Edition of the Mahābhārata*. Pune: Bhandarkar Oriental Research Institute.